The Secret Healer's Aromatherapy Eczema Treatment.

The Professional Aromatherapist's Guide to Healing Eczema, Itchy Skin Rashes and Atopic Dermatitis with Essential Oils and Holistic Medicine.

All Rights Reserved. No part of this publication may be reproduced in any form or by any means, including scanning, photocopying, or otherwise without prior written permission of the copyright holder.

Copyright © 2014 Elizabeth Ashley – The Secret Healer

Introduction

In the United States 31.6 million people are reported to have eczema. In the UK the figures are harder to come by. Reports from 2009 show a 40% increase in reported cases of eczema over the last five years. The University of Nottingham made projections from their findings and predicted that by 2014 as many as 457.26 per 1000 people will report having eczema at sometime in their lives. That means for every 2.19 people you meet, one of them is a potential customer for you. Do you often meet .19 of a person? No, nor me. Let's round it up. To be conservative, write the words "**a potential market of one in three people**" into your business plan.

The health authority tells us too, these patients will visit the doctors four times, each year, about their skin. Sufferers are eager to improve their skin conditions and those figures suggest they are happy to keep working at it until they achieve their objective. Let me ask you, reader, can you accommodate a few patients whom you can rely upon to consistently book appointments at least once every three months? I thought you might!

To begin with: a warning, then. The internet is bursting at the seams with professionals declaring aromatherapy won't help eczema. Page after page of opinions are spun off one single research paper which cites massage with essential oils as further aggravating eczematous conditions. Let me start by saying, I agree. Massage is not the best course of action. But that does not negate the use of essential oils. There are other, far better ways to use them.

How about in creams and lotions, for instance?

Waiting rooms across the world are abuzz with chatter about the new cream doctors are giving their patients. Surveys across the NHS state this salve, **licensed, patented and trademarked by a recognised drug company** is the most popular course of eczema treatment with patients. Interestingly, it's made of plant extracts. Actually, it's **made from an essential oil**.

Meanwhile, in Japan, groundbreaking discoveries have uncovered a vital common denominator in children with atopic eczema (the allergic kind). We now know sufferers of atopic eczema have a far higher likelihood of having non-alcoholic fatty liver disease. Scientists in India answered this discovery by running clinical trials to see if plant essences can help this particular problem. They chose an essence any decent aromatherapist would have quickly offered as a solution. Guess what? It's worked. Ginger shows early signs of treating this fatty liver problem, which is believed not only be behind atopic eczema, but allergies in general as well as myriad other health complaints.

This is not the first time plant medicine has played an important part in a medical breakthrough. Digitalis, Morphine and Valium are just a handful of drugs which started off their lives in the herbal healer's tool box. The pharmaceutical industry will take years to patent the drugs they create from the findings cited in this paper. These trials from the labs, show essential oils attacking pathogens in petri dishes, sadly on rats too, but also in human trials. They prove aromatherapy not only is effective, but has answers far ahead of its time. You simply have to know where to look for them. The thing is too, I bet you have most of the plants they recommend in your oils box.

This book takes the wisdom of my Advanced Aromatherapy Diploma (studied in 1994) and matches it to the findings of the today's conventional medicine research. Not only are many of the oils we were taught to use, and those found to be effective in a lab, identical; the sheer potency of the results the scientists are finding is startling.

There is very little here I did not know back in the 90s. My step father Michael Cook and my mum Jill Bruce were travelling the country at exhibitions doling out pots of cream helping literally thousands of people. The repeat orders, over 30 years, have attested to how well their treatments have worked. Now though, those early beginnings of fringe science are gathering momentum, gaining speed, pushing that ancient and sacred wisdom right into the limelight of the masses. You know where you will find it in less than ten years time? On those shelves behind the pharmacist's counter!

As qualified healing professionals you owe it to yourselves, and aromatherapy, to benefit from this before the drug companies do. What's more no matter how cleverly they refine the active ingredients to treat these complaints, holistic medicine will always treat it better. Don't get me wrong, I love going to my doctor as much as the next hypochondriac, but he can only give me a 15 minute appointment.

The extra time you give your patient to learn their treatment and understand their dis-ease is vital, the space you can allow them to relax into who they want to be, and that quietness to let the illness leave their bodies...they won't find that in the doctor's waiting room, but they should with you.

Never mind us though, what about those patients who **need** your help. Think about the salesman who struggles to make his quota of sales because people worry they will catch that rash he has all over his face. Consider how you could change the life of the mother who has to listen to her child screaming in agony all through the night. Think of the relief you bring to the child who has spent their entire life itching, scratching and bleeding even, from their weeping and angry skin.

Whilst this book is written by an aromatherapist, for aromatherapists, it covers a whole range of therapies because I agree with the doctors; aromatherapy can't do this alone. On the surface we can **reduce the itching**, **heal the cuts** and abrasions and **calm the redness**, but there is *so much more*.

Living with eczema is like a house of cards, one false move and the whole lot comes crashing down around you. Maybe your patient ate the wrong food, picked up some animal hair on their clothes or even got upset....sometimes the house stays standing, other times, their eczema detonates. It is imperative you strengthen the foundations and treat the illness from the root up.

- Learn to cleanse the liver of debris causing flare ups.

- Witness the strange connection between the mind and the skin. Just what are the emotions causing eczema? You'll be amazed how simple a correlation that can be.

- Discover why the stomach holds the key to eczema treatment.

- Activate the body's internal healing systems using the acupressure points clinically proven to help eczema.

- Expose skeletal misalignments exacerbating the problem.

- Uncover the secret combination of essential oils found, in laboratory conditions, to eradicate *candida albacans.*

- Learn how hypnosis can recondition the mind's responses to the condition. I'll show you how to get your hands on a specially designed recording for less than a trip to the 99 cents store. You'll be amazed how powerfully it works.

- Download a set of beautifully illustrated charts to help you make the most of the chiropractic, acupressure, vitamin therapy and even chakra healing. I'm giving you this free when you buy this book.

- Uncover a whole new approach to eczema treatment. I promise you, your healing will never be the same again.

Table of Contents

Introduction 3
Table of Contents 9
About the Author 12
How to use this book 14
    What is eczema 17
    The main types of eczema 18
    The dysfunction of the skin 22
    Atopy 24
    Atopic or allergic march 24
    The importance of the liver 27
    The house of cards 29
    Metabolic disorders 30
    Allergies 31
    Leaky gut syndrome 33
    Candida 33
    Parasites 37
    Geopathic stress 39
    Where to pin the eczema source 41
Chapter 2 The Psychological Triggers of Eczema 43
    The emotions causing eczema 43
    Trauma 47
Chapter 3 Eczema and Diet 52
    Food combinations 52

Magnesium	56
Calcium	58
Copper	59
Zinc	60
Iron	61
Choline	62
Biotin	63
Determine Food Allergies	64
Subtle Energies	69
Chiropractic	70
The Meridians	75
Acupressure for eczema	76
Essential oil therapy	79
Bases	80
Baths	81
Showers	81
Carrier Oils	81
Essential Oils	83
To stop itching	83
To treat the surface eczema	84
To heal broken skin	85
To reduce scarring	87
Anti allergenic	87

Circulation for varicose eczema 87
To cleanse the liver 87
Hepatic oils 87
Fatty Liver 88
To cleanse heavy metal debris 88
The adrenals 89
Digestive cleansers 89
Kidneys 89
Gall bladder 89
Spleen 90
Parasites 90
    Blood 90
    Tissues 91
    Vermifuge 91
    Excreted toxins 91
    Insect bites 91
Candida albacans & Malessezzia furfur 92
Geopathic stress 93
Oils for the emotions 93
Oils for the chakras 95
Conclusion 103
Other works by the author 106
Bibliography 117
Disclaimer 126

About the Author

Elizabeth Ashley qualified as an aromatherapist in 1993, and then passed her Advanced Aromatherapy Diploma in 1994. She has been practicing aromatherapy for almost 21 years.

In 1999, she fell into a whole new career in the aggressive commercial sector of recruitment consultancy. There she discovered her father's second hand car salesman genes had passed along and found she had quite a gift of the gab! More than that, she discovered she could sell...and then some.

In 2008, Elizabeth fell ill during pregnancy with a blood clot in her lungs. The pulmonary embolism prevented her from working and she started to write. Very quickly she gained her first contract as a ghost writer...a recipe book for cheese cakes!

In 2010 she was published professionally for her work on Galbanum oil in the Aromatherapy Thymes, journal of the International Federation of Aromatherapists, and on Tuberose oil by the New Zealand Register of Holistic Therapist.

In 2011 she was seconded on a consultative basis to Walsall Independent Treatment Centre, designed to be a rainbow bridge between traditional and complementary medicines. There she became aware of the rumblings of change in healthcare. Her book *Sales Strategies for Gentle Souls* explains the connotations of this.

In 2014 she ranks in the top 50 contract writers on the freelancer marketplace Elance.com. She is the ghost writer of seven number one Amazon best sellers in the natural healing category. She lives in Shropshire with her husband and youngest son, kept company by their cat, the budgie and many shoals of tropical fish! Her elder son and daughter attend university and make her prouder than anything ever could.

Elizabeth Ashley is The Secret Healer. Her books are designed to fill gaps in aromatherapy knowledge and train therapists, to bring their business into the cyber age and make their practices excel.

How to use this book

This book is a manual. I have created it in a way I feel it is easy to just dip in and find out what you need to know. It is separated into physical, then mental, then nutrition and food, then spiritual.

The physical part is very scientific, but easy to follow. I have deliberately sliced everything down into bite sized chunks. This book *Aromatherapy Eczema Treatment* is part of a set, designed to be like lessons all hanging off each other. Throughout, I refer to other books in **The Secret Healer** series. This is to avoid repetition of the same subjects over and over in each book. Each one has its specific focus. Whilst this is about eczema, I also talk a lot about identifying food intolerances, how allergies come about, candida and parasites, all of which can play a part in eczema, but also in other conditions too.

There are two of my other books, specifically, that will help you here. *The Professional Stress Solution* will help you to tackle the stress related, flare up aspect and *The Essential Oils Liver Cleanse* will help you understand some of the emotional aspects of the disease as well as actually helping you to clean up their liver dysfunction too. As with all complementary medicine learning, I think, the more you know, the more you discover you don't know. The journey gets ever longer. These two books, however, should help you a lot. Consider these to be step by step stages through the maze dis-ease can be.

You will notice I write dis-ease as a hyphenated word often through the text. This is deliberate. This, points to the fact I suspect the subject is indicative of the spirit being ill at ease. It might also refer to their emotions. Either way, the illness has come from their spiritual or emotional dis-ease.

Feel free to read as much or as little of the book as you like. The essential oils are listed separately at the back, in the last chapter. You may just want to jump ahead to those and I won't be too offended!

Other resources available to you:

There are no pictures in this book. Instead I supply beautifully detailed drawings for you to print off and add to each case history you do. I find patients feel more reassured by you presenting the relevant chart than hunting through a book. At each relevant point in the book, I shall post a link for you to download and print. There are charts available to show: misalignments of the spine, acupressure points on meridians, nutritional therapy and the chakras.

Are you ready then?

Let's do it!

What is eczema

In some ways that is a bit like asking, what is a dog?! Breeds of dogs tend to look very different, sound different and will react in any number of different ways. Eczema is very much the same.

The absolute "must – have" criterion is:

There must be itchy skin.

You should also be able to find three or probably more pointers from the following list:

- The skin is dry
- It flakes
- There is redness
- It might be blistered
- It might break open and bleed
- Eczema is visible on the limbs, especially at the flexures of the joints, on the cheeks or forehead
- Redness and itching in the folds of the elbows and knees as well as on the neck
- Symptoms will often show themselves as early as a 2 years old
- There might also be a family history of eczema, allergies or asthma

Eczema is not contagious. You cannot catch it by touching someone's skin. It *is* however hereditary and there will often be trends of it in a family. It has its roots in allergic reaction. You have a 20% chance of developing eczema if your parents had it. If both were sufferers that number increases to between 50-80% likelihood.

The main types of eczema

- Contact dermatitis

- Seborrheic Eczema

- Discoid Eczema

- Varicose Eczema (also known as Gravitational or statis eczema)

- Eczema cracquelée (also known sometimes as Asteatotic eczema)

- Atopic eczema

You will also come across two other skin disorders, these are dermatitis and psoriasis. Psoriasis is not the same as eczema, and will be covered in a book of its own in 2015. Dermatitis is the same as eczema, however not all dermatitis is eczematous. That sounds terribly confusing but, put simply, dermatitis means there is an inflammation of the skin. This can happen because you have touched something that either causes the reaction, or causes an allergy that causes a reaction. Keep reading....it will become easier to understand.

Contact Dermatitis

In the main, this is work related. It can range from mild irritation to full scale chemical burning. It has developed because the patient has touched a chemical repeatedly, for example a hairdresser with peroxide. The main irritants responsible for this are:

Weak irritants, for example, diluted acids, diluted alkalis, solvents, soaps, detergents, metallic salts, cement, resins and cutting fluids. These are the commonest, but not only, causes of irritant contact dermatitis.

Seborrhoeic Eczema

This condition tends to start on the scalp as dandruff, then redness and irritation turns to increased scaling.

It usually begins on the scalp, then wanders down the neck until it develops in the eyebrows, down the folds at the side of the nose, the face and the temples. The red flaking can be particularly troublesome behind the ears, where the greasy flakes get stuck in the patient's hair. If it finds its way into the ears and ear canal, it is called ear eczema, funnily enough. You might also find it in the folds under the breasts, armpits, groin and between the buttocks. These are sweaty areas, basically, because the eczema is caused by a reaction of the sebaceous glands.

Recent research has found a type of yeast is present on the skin called *pityrosporum ovale,* otherwise known as *malessezzia furfur*. We cover this in more detail in the section about *candida albacans* which is another spore.

Discoid Eczema

This red coin-shaped eczema tends to develop on the lower leg, the trunk and the forearms. It is also known as nummular dermatitis. Mainly it is an adult's affliction, but teenagers and children do sometimes get it too.

The surface of the breakout becomes very bumpy. The patches ooze, get very itchy and encrusted. Then as the surface scales they simply become dry and flaky.

Varicose Eczema (also known as Gravitational or statis eczema)

Varicose eczema tends to affect mainly women, later on in their lives. It can happen if they have had a blood clot in their legs, have varicose veins or if they are overweight.

In these situations, circulation can't move the fluid up the body fast enough and so it pools down at the ankles causing them to swell, putting pressure on the vein walls. Over time, the skin becomes very thin and fragile and on some occasions can ulcerate, breaking open and leaving holes in the patient's leg.

Eczema cracquelée (also known sometimes as Asteatotic eczema)

This predominately happens to people over the age of 60. The cause is as yet, undetermined. It is thought it might be due to a decrease of oils in the skin as they age and possibly low humidity might have a bearing too. Taking baths that are too hot and generally over-cleansing definitely makes this condition worse. It tends to look like crazy paving and break into fissures. Luckily, these are usually only surface level and are not really dangerous lesions in themselves, but clearly infection is a consideration here.

Atopic eczema or Atopic Dermatitis

This is an allergic eczema which we will cover more in depth in a moment. Both terms relate to the same condition.

In medical journals you will see eczema referred to as Atopic Dermatitis or AD. You will also see **contact dermatitis** where the skin has come into contact with an **external irritant**. **Atopic dermatitis** is more concerned with **internal irritation**. When we look at atopic dermatitis in more depth in a moment, it is very easy to see the difference between the two.

In eczema, the skin flakes away or becomes damaged in some way. Let's start by looking at the dermatology element of the disease first.

The dysfunction of the skin

Here, I would like to take the opportunity to recommend a book to you I did not write. I do, however think it is quite wonderful. The Eczema Diet by Karen Fischer shines like a star in the brightest sky of healing books. I wish I had written it, or at least could get hold of her to tell her how great it is, but I seem not to be able to. I have used it extensively in the research for this book, but you should read definitely read her book too. She cites the work of Professor Michael Cork from the dermatology department of the University of Sheffield to show the breakdown of the skin and I am going to do the same.

Imagine the skin cells as bricks in a very large structure. These bricks would need to be held together by iron rods to strengthen the support. In your skin, these iron rods are binders called *corneodesmosomes*. The mortar, holding the bricks together, is molecules containing waxes and fats called lipids.

Consider then, with eczema the skin barrier is thinner than it would normally be. These iron rods no longer have adequate protection from external forces at work. It's a bit like the roof is off the construction now and so these iron rods are cast open to the elements. With no barrier covering, they deteriorate and eventually they snap. Now in eczema, this is exactly what happens. The corneodesmosomes snap too early causing this flaking of the skin that we see. The lipids also crack and so there is this perpetual breakdown of the skin. It crumbles and of course, this compromises the barrier even more. Infection can get into the cracks and abrasions, but also allergens and irritants can too. As well as making the allergic reaction worse this also perpetuates the flaking. A never ending circle of skin breakage continues.

The skin *should* also naturally be slightly acidic in order to make it difficult for fungi, bacteria and all other kinds of lovelies to grow. This layer is called the Acid Mantle. It should sit with a ph of around 5.5, but in people with eczema, (seborrhoeic eczema in particular) this ph tends to be less acidic. Because of this, there are no defences against allergens such as dust mites, cat hairs etc. We will also see malessezzia fungal break outs.

Atopy

Earlier I mentioned Atopic Dermatitis. The word *atopy* is from the Greek word which means *special, unusual* or *out of place*. It pertains to hypersensitivity with allergens. An atopic disorder will only flare if someone comes into contact with a certain allergen…there must be a catalyst.

But a catalyst will not cause a reaction on its own. In the case of eczema, an allergic reaction happens because of a high level of antibodies in the system called IgE antibodies. *Immunoglobulin E* binds allergens to mast cells and causes inflammation by releasing histamine into the blood stream. Everyone has these antibodies in small numbers but for some people they work particularly aggressively.

Atopic or allergic march

Many of you will be aware doctors agree there is a link between eczema, allergic rhinitis and asthma. Often, this is can have a familial link, but not always, although it does influence the chances this link will occur.

Doctors call this relationship the *atopic march* or the *allergic march*. The march follows certain steps and can be influenced by many external factors which determines the severity of the illness that develops. The presence of IgE antibodies means eczema will often develop into allergic rhinitis (the most recognised form of this is hay fever) and then to asthma.

In the bibliography I have attached a reference to a brilliant paper called "The Atopic March" which brings together the findings of an inordinate number of studies, but here are the edited highlights. The abbreviation AD is used extensively, standing for Atopic Dermatitis.

The International Studies of Asthma and Allergies in Childhood revealed statistics detailing incidences of Atopic Dermatitis varied from 0.3% to 20.5% between countries. This is a massive variation. Across the board though, every country showed their problems of AD had grown *consistently* over time. In the UK between 2001 - 2005, incidences were rising by 38 people per 1000 every year.

I'll use US statistics here for ease, because they seem to be more transparent in the data, but remember the correlations between data remain the same for every country. Remember too, this part pertains to Atopic Eczema (relating to allergens) but that is not the only type of eczema there is. This bit is about <u>eczema caused by allergies</u>.

In the US 17.9% of 5-9 year old children suffers from eczema.

- 45% of those first presented with symptoms in the first 6 months of their lives
- 60% of those in the first year
- 85% by their 5th year.

- Less than half of these incidences had been resolved by their 7th birthdays.
- 60% of them would have resolution by adult hood.

So we know then, the first five years of a child's life is critical in terms of allergic response.

AD is also seen as a major risk factor in <u>*asthma*</u> because of the levels of IgE antibodies in the system. IgE antibodies cause environmental allergies. It has been discovered when these are found to be present in children aged between 2-4 years old they are at higher risk of progressing through the march than those without IgE sensitisation.

It is approximated that 70% of patients with *severe* AD develop asthma compared with 20-30% with *mild* AD but only 8% of the general population.

To throw a spanner in the works though, whilst <u>studies show there is a direct link between eczema and childhood asthma</u>, a separate cohort study of 22 year olds, found there is <u>not a link between eczema and **adult** asthma</u>.

It is not clearly understood why some children will grow out of their AD and others will not. Science agrees genetics and environmental factors seem to have an influence. What is so far undetermined is what exactly that entails and studies continue to examine how this may be influenced.

Findings show the ratio for the risk of developing asthma with AD compared to the risk without it is a massive 2.14. *Twice as likely.* The Tuscon Children's Respiratory Study also showed that 18% of six year olds with persistent wheezing problems had had eczema by the time they were two.

To sum all of this up then: allergies play a massive part.

The importance of the liver

The skin is the largest organ in the body. In second place in terms of size, comes the liver. It is responsible for a number of functions to do with keeping the skin healthy. Firstly it looks after the condition of the blood and it helps the body remove waste products. It takes away fats, toxins and also pharmaceutical products and then it sends them to the excretory system to get rid of. It also takes nutrients absorbed from foods and makes them into amino acids for the body to regenerate and repair itself.

Research, done at the beginning of the millennium, in Japan, showed some rather unsettling results...albeit extremely illuminating.

When tested in the year 2000, a group of non-obese children were tested for fatty livers by an ultrasound scan. 17.6% of the children with atopic dermatitis had fatty livers compared with only 3.2% of non atopic children. Then in 2001-3, the prevalence was studied further and was found to be increasing annually. In 2001, it reached 12.5% in non-atopic children, 13.1% in patients with bronchial asthma, 13.7% in patients with allergic rhinitis, or 33.9% in patients with atopic dermatitis, in 2003.

To recap for a moment: Scientists agree non-alcoholic liver disease is on the rise (this applies in adults as well as children, by the way). They also agree AD is on the rise. Further, they confirm AD is directly linked to fatty liver.

For a change, allopathic medicine and complementary medicine agree on the next point. This area of research must be well funded and transparent over the next few years, because this decline in health will influence future healthcare spending on a global scale. This fatty liver dimension naturally does not only have implications for skin care, but also for obesity, metabolic syndrome, heart attacks and strokes to name but a few.

Many things affect the liver to make it fatty. Diet is known to be a factor, alcohol, medicines, fertilizers, even wi-fi might have a bearing if some sources are to be believed! I cover it in far more in depth in the *Essential Oil Liver Cleanse*, but as you can see the correlation to liver is there, the rise in incidences is there, and I'd be silly not to point out...there are potentially more and more patients out there!

A quick overview though:

If the truth be told, most peoples' livers' are struggling. I describe it as running a car for 10,000 miles and then putting diesel into it instead of the correct petrol. It takes just one trigger for it all to go terribly wrong.

We eat over processed foods with very little nutritional content. Antibiotics such as erythromycin wipe out vitamin B. This is the fuel the liver runs on. Most of our food is treated with fertilisers and petrochemicals and the liver does not know how to get rid of them. (Explained more fully in *Essential Oil Liver Cleanse*)

Then, we have stress responses. When you get angry or upset your adrenal glands kick into gear raising blood pressure, heart rate and breathing. It floods the body with hormones, which over time, start to poison the body. The adrenals are fuelled by glucocorticoids which are made by the liver and so, after a while, the liver becomes utterly exhausted by the stress. (Explained more fully in *The Professional Stress Solution.*)

The house of cards

What determines if a person will get eczema or not then? Ugh, where on earth shall we start?! You will definitely have this weird IgE thing going on. This may or many not have been inherited from mom or dad. But probably, it was.

So then the IgE finds an allergen and hitches a ride on it which may or may not cause a flare up. Some days it will, some days it won't, and some days it may end up with a hospital stay.

I like to think of it like a house of cards. The status quo of an eczema sufferer is *always* precarious at best. One day though, just a single card too many is placed on top and the whole thing comes tumbling down. We'll call this the joker in the pack. As the book unfolds you will see, if the joker had been placed in a different spot at a different time, he would not have bought the house down.

Metabolic disorders

For the most part you are going to find the excretory systems being compromised in eczema too. All this toxicity puts pressure on the primary ones: these are the bowels, kidneys and liver. They then transfer pressure to the secondary elimination channels, the skin (in eczema) and the lungs (in asthma).

In the stomach, we also usually find there are low levels of hydrochloric acid (HCA). This is secreted by the lining of the stomach when we eat food. Its job is to initiate proteins and fats. It encourages bile flow and pancreatic juices.

When the acid is strong it inhibits harmful bacteria, it kills diseases and eradicates parasites in food. It also affects absorption of vitamins. When levels of HCA are too low, the body cannot assimilate calcium, zinc, iron, magnesium, copper, and vitamins B and C. As ever, in complementary medicine, there is a catch 22. The body also *requires* vitamin B6 and zinc to produce HCA!

Signals of this happening shows in the fingernails. Vertical ridging shows malnutrition through low levels of HCA. With no proteins to help build the construction of the nail, ridges form.

Allergies

The Department of Food Allergies at Stanford University offers the following guidelines.

- 38% of individuals with a single allergy will go on to develop multiple allergies.

- Food allergies get worse if exposures are sporadic.

- The following eight foods account for 90% of all food allergies: milk, egg, peanut, tree nuts, fish, shellfish, soy and wheat.

- It is possible to grow out of an allergy and the chance of growing out of a food allergy does not depend on how many allergies a patient has. There is a 20% chance of outgrowing allergies to peanuts, tree nuts and shellfish and a 75% chance of outgrowing allergies to milk, eggs, soy, fish, and wheat.

- Reactions to allergens can alter. There is a 25% chance of a person having a completely different reaction the next time they are exposed to his or her allergen.

- An allergic reaction to food can affect the skin, the gastrointestinal tract, the respiratory tract and, in the most serious cases, the cardiovascular system. Reactions can range from mild to the severe and potentially life-threatening condition known as anaphylaxis.

- Mild symptoms may include one or more of the following: hives (reddish, swollen, itchy areas on the skin); eczema (a persistent dry, itchy rash); an itchy mouth; nausea or vomiting; diarrhoea; abdominal pain; and nasal congestion or a runny nose.

- Many people think the terms food allergy and food intolerance are the same thing. However, they are not. Food intolerance, unlike a food allergy, doesn't involve the immune system and they are not life-threatening. Having trouble digesting the milk sugar lactose, Lactose intolerance, is an example of this. Symptoms include abdominal cramps, bloating and diarrhoea. **A food**

32

allergy occurs when the immune system reacts to a certain food.

- To the best of their knowledge, the rate of sibling allergies is about 60%

- The factors that can influence who will develop an allergy and who won't are: Smoking, pollution and genetics.

Leaky gut syndrome

This is more related to food allergies and intolerance, but not exclusively. Over time, as the body keeps reacting to allergens, the tissues become inflamed. If this happens repeatedly, after a while the cells actually physically separate from each other by moving apart. This creates holes. We call this membrane permeability; it almost becomes like Swiss cheese, random holes all over. This allows food to leak through into the blood stream. Unable to go through the regular excretory channels, the skin tries to take a turn, but cannot cope with such a systemic overload. Again, we have the potential for eczema, and in fact psoriasis, flare ups here.

Candida

Foods may be working as allergens and so cleansing the digestive tract is vital. But it is not only food which can be the problem. Candida is also likely to be a protagonist. Research shows 70% of patients with AD also have *candida albicans* overgrowth in the gut.

Candida is a yeast organism which lives in all of us. It is supposed to be there. In its correct amounts and, in the right environment, candida is a friend. Usually the immune system and the helpful bacteria in the gut keep its levels in check, but when they begin to rise, the yeast releases harmful toxins into the colon. These toxins can cause a whole host of problems from migraines, bladder inflammations and especially skin eruptions. More obvious symptoms are oral and vaginal thrush and nappy rash.

It is perfectly common for a child to be born with thrush in their mouths too. The yeast infection is in the mother's birth canal and baby picks it up. The doctor very quickly spots this and they tend to treat symptoms either with the allopathic treatment nystatin or the complementary and gentler option Caprystatin. Both are very effective treatments, the problem is they will also wipe out the good bacterial flora too. Consequently we now also have a metabolic problem. We will talk about that in a moment.

Just for a second let's think about vaginal thrush (anybody would think it was tea time, that always seems to be the time the TV think I want to know about it in the ad breaks). What is it usually coupled with? Cystitis, right? The doc gives you cream to get rid of the thrush, then you get cystitis and he gives you antibiotics. That wipes the vitamin B out, and so the bacteria can't be regulated and your old friend thrush is singing from your knickers again. I'll bet you didn't miss him either. Some women suffer this cycle for years.

The way to eradicate candida, sadly is diet. I say sadly because the relevant diet is so strict. It wipes out anything acidic or sugary off the menu as well as fermented food and fungi. Again we'll cross that bridge later but for a moment I want to talk about the sugar issue. Candida albacans loves sugar. Remember candida is a yeast, and what does yeast need to be activated? You got it...sugar.

I stood aghast yesterday when I was thinking about how to put this part of the book together to make it easy to understand (because candida can be a minefield) and I walked into the kitchen to the most incredible smell of bread. For a moment I though my husband had found a domestic streak, but then I realised the smell was not bread...it was yeast. He uses it to feed the plants CO_2 in the fish tank to make them grow faster.

In the sink, was a glass full of freshly prepared yeast, bubbling, fizzing, rising at a fervent pace, threatening to overspill and fill my sink. As I watched, it made me realise why yeast attacks are so fierce. The speed it moved was phenomenal and that happens in your gut! But yeast needs its catalyst for the reaction. Sugar. And how does it get that? It sets up a craving and you dive for the mars bar.

More saliently....when does it set up the worst cravings? PMS, migraines...here are your candida problems. If there are sugar cravings, suspect there may be candida. How depressing, this means the very thing you think is making you feel better is the blasted thing making you ill!!!

You must watch your patient's diet to try to ascertain whether there are cravings. Asking your patient to keep a detailed food diary will help you to do this. I would also definitely recommend making a glass of yeast to watch the reaction and anchor in your mind just how fast yeast works.

Now, think back to right at the beginning of the book. Can you remember I said seborrheic eczema also had a yeast spore? *Malessezzia furfur* is treated in exactly the same manner as candida.

Just as an aside, Candida often has an underlying parasite. (You thought the thrush was the best I can come up with at the dinner table....oh no, it gets far worse!) It is thought that the parasites excrete into our systems and that upsets the flora balance setting off a yeast attack.

I know I sound like an 8 year old girl in the school yard but, gross! (We used to cross our fingers and shout "Eew get barley" when something was that revolting, did you?)

Parasites

Revoltingly, many of us are unwittingly playing host to unwanted visitors. There are the obvious ones like tape worm and round worm but, also, there can be horrid parasites from insect bites.

Actually if you do your job carefully, eczema flare ups with their roots in these nasties are quite easy to spot.

Here's what you'll hear as they gleefully shove some unsightly limb in your face...

"Have a look at this! Bet you've never seen anything like that before! The doctor's given me all sorts but it always seems to come back. The strange thing is it only flares up when it's hot!"(Or may be cold on some occasions but the key is the seasonal cycle).

From there try and trace back how long they have had the problem. You can usually match it to a holiday. They have been attacked by some horrid fly (often in response to being stepped on in the sand) which of course they may or may not remember. When they have come home it has been too cold for the parasite, so it has lain dormant until the sun came out.

This is when you see the horrid skin lesions. Incidentally, I have also seen this happen from building sand and farm yard manure too. I actually think I picked one up years ago when I was licked by some kind of deer thing at the Safari Park and I had an open wound on my hand. The flies get in, they attack, but the patient has no idea until the insect's natural cycle recommences.

A more mundane source can be eating raw salad and fruit which has not been washed and of course, the one we all know: uncooked pork. Another clue which might lead you to believe there is a digestive parasite in particular is ravenous hunger. Just as the cat never stops mewling for food when she has a worm, humans respond in just the same way.

Isn't that delightful? Never mind how revolting it is, I'm absolutely certain you'll do a celebratory dance next time someone shows you their scabby hand!

I am being rather flippant about it because frankly it is vile, but the affects of parasitic infection are dreadful really. Not only could it be eczema you see, but PMS is a big one, cystitis, diarrhoea, asthma, and psoriasis too.

In the words of my Advanced Aromatherapy course notes since I have never found a better phrase: Parasites lead to an insidious breakdown of health.

Nutri- West make a very good product called Par-X which is very effective in dealing with mal nutrition caused by parasitic invasion.

Geopathic stress

When I trained back in the early 90s, this was taken as read. Architects across the world were issuing scathing statements about Sick Building Syndrome. A report in the early 80s had blamed many conditions on poor ventilation in buildings. It came to be synonymous with open plan offices, but also council high rises.

In 2006 however, a Swedish investigate recommended Sick Building Syndrome should no longer be used as a possible diagnosis, but most practitioners would agree the theory does still hold water. Even the NHS feel it is a valid explanation for illness in people who work in libraries, schools and museums, that is open plan environments which house many, many people.

The NHS page on Sick Building Syndrome says:

"The symptoms of SBS may include:

- headaches and dizziness
- nausea (feeling sick)
- aches and pains

- fatigue (extreme tiredness)
- poor concentration
- shortness of breath or chest tightness
- eye and throat irritation
- irritated, blocked or running nose
- skin irritation (skin rashes, dry itchy skin)

The symptoms of SBS can appear on their own, or in combination with each other, and they may vary from day to day. Different individuals in the same building may have different symptoms. They usually improve or disappear altogether after leaving the building."

Wow, some of those are looking familiar, don't you think?

Sources then, it relates

"Possible risk factors for SBS may include:

- poor ventilation
- low humidity
- high temperature or changes in temperature throughout the day

- airborne particles, such as dust, carpet fibres or fungal spores

- airborne chemical pollutants, such as those from cleaning materials or furniture, or ozone produced by photocopiers and printers

- physical factors, such as electrostatic charges

- poor standards of cleanliness in the working environment

- poor lighting that causes glare or flicker on visual display units (VDUs)

- improper use of display screen equipment

- psychological factors, such as stress or low staff morale

Many of these you will recognise as reactions to allergies, spores (see candida), possible liver reactions to positive ions and electromagnetism.

Where to pin the eczema source

It's fair to say eczema is always swinging between catalysts. Its cause might be 50% down to genetics, 40% to allergies and 10% down to emotional state on the day. That is to say, you can blame washing powder, tomatoes and next door's cat, (or permutations of the three) but your mood will also play a part in determining whether a flare might occur. Let's give our brains a break from allergies for a moment and have a think about emotions.

Chapter 2 The Psychological Triggers of Eczema

The emotions causing eczema

What we are going to find here, is some days a person will have skin that is better than others. Most sufferers will agree their ill health will coincide with periods of stress, but not always. For many sufferers, it can be difficult to comprehend the connection between anxiety and the skin. Between the two, however, is the interface of the nervous system. The base of the subcutaneous layer of the skin is riddled with nerve endings endlessly relaying messages about the emotions out to the outside world.

What is one of the most obvious outward signs of emotional discomfort? We blush when we are embarrassed – a direct link from the emotional response to the outward signs on the skin. The messages run straight from the brain to the nerve endings in the skin and trigger the capillaries to act.

You should be clear there, is always this interplay between the mind and the emotions and the physical health of a person. How they feel about their life and circumstances will often be behind their outward symptoms. There are certain emotions associated with internal organs these are:

- Liver - Anger

- Heart- Irritation
- Lungs - Grief
- Kidneys- Fear
- Spleen – Worry

Those of you who have read any of my other books, by now, I hope are thinking about emotions which might set this off. Full marks to those who have thought anger, because it pertains to the liver but....with eczema there is often a very certain aspect to the anger. It is directed inwards, toward the sufferer themselves.

The interesting thing here is we have an outward manifestation of the internal processing...it's on the skin for everyone to see. Now the emotional aspects of the skin are how we present ourselves to the world; or maybe more accurately how *we* think the world perceives *us*.

The main emotional factors underlying eczema pertain to hurt personality or individuality. We can say also sense of insecurity and perfectionism.

In some ways the emotional aspects of eczema are very sad to think about. You are likely to see outward manifestations of suppressed emotions because the child so desperately wants to be seen as good. Perhaps as a child they haven't wanted to shout "look at me" when the focus has been on another child, and they have pushed that anger down...because frankly they are a nice kid and they feel it's the right thing to do.

If you don't over think it, this mind body association is quite easy to grasp. It is about irritation...with one's self. The patient's nagging doubt they are not quite good enough....or they think *other people* might think they are not good enough. This endless need to get better and better at things, or even act perfectly, often underlies the outward irritation. You get this perfectionism element to the personality but of course, the more they want to act and look perfect, the more they see themselves as failing because they can't sit still for scratching the rash. This makes me think of another one of these weird linguistic correlations. What do you call someone who can't keep to their decisions, or is unreliable? How strange that the eczema sufferer is likely to be annoyed at their self for being....flaky... when they can't resist the need to scratch!

The emotion behind eczema is very much about frustration, feeling they can't express themselves fully, always worried they will be seen as not good-enough...and of course they can come to hate themselves for that. Addressing the emotions of eczema is vital. They will feel self conscious, frustrated and angry about their skin, but weirdly those emotions may have been the joker in their pack of cards...even before the rash appeared.

Referring back to what I said in the last chapter: "The status quo of an eczema sufferer is *always* precarious at best." Put yourself, for a moment, into the shoes of the parent of a child with eczema. There is this constant watching of the environment for allergens. There is the fear that scratching will break the skin, and always worry about what might send their child into tears of agony again. So the child is watched, it has to be careful, it has to conform, comply, act in the correct safest way….and so the emotional cycle continues, because as soon as they have a breakout they feel like they have let their parent down. What a terribly insecure way to live. Insecurity…and the cycle spirals on…..

There can be a slightly more malevolent dimension to the emotions of eczema though; entirely subconsciously, of course. A skin disorder can be a most manipulative tool. The worse your skin is, the more attention you are likely to get. You have this dynamic of the victim also becoming the victimiser…because it does impose a certain amount of power. It's not deliberate, there will be likely no conscious awareness of it, but the spirit can be a little demon when it wants to be.

At this point, I will say in *The Professional Stress Solution* I talk about a Traditional Chinese Medicine phenomena called Yin Disease. I would urge you to read this because it will help you with how the emotions affect a person's demeanour and health. There are two salient points relevant here though. A person with yin disease (in which, eczema plays its part because it is stress related illness) happily sees themselves as a victim. It's also important to note their tissues disintegrate....here's your flaky skin.

I will add here, that I do actually feel very strongly that a person with a rash all over their body is damn right: they are a victim and I feel very sorry for them. *My* opinion, about their status, however, is not important. It is how they see *themselves,* that is...and it is making their own health worse. This is another emotional dimension, as therapists we need to address.

Trauma

Going back to that house of cards again, the text book case of an eczema suffer is they develop a rash between about 2-4, it may or may not develop into hay fever and asthma. But....

Why might a rash suddenly appear outside of this "normal" Atopic march? What might happen to a child of 5, for instance, that might suddenly determine they have itchy legs?

More often than not, this can be traced back to a single traumatic event. Again there is more about this is the Essential Oil Liver Cleanse (because traumatic events affect the liver

47

primarily). The trauma might be emotional, but it could also be physical too,

This really is where contact dermatitis comes in. I suffered a really bad insect bite once, which badly scarred my leg. This is one of my worst affected eczema sites. Many of the patients you are likely to see will have eczema on their hands from handling some kind of chemical. Most obvious examples are nurses who wash their hands incessantly, farmers who handle chemicals for the farm, hairdressers who handle colorants and peroxides.

You have this physical assault on the skin from the chemicals, but they also absorb through the skin (and / or are inhaled). They enter the blood stream. The body tries to assimilate them, which it can do to a certain extent, but in the final processes they cannot be metabolised and they lodge in the liver. And round we go again!

You see? I told you it gets easier...just always look at the liver.

And the adrenals!

Let's have a little test here. Do you know what medication the doctor will give you to put onto eczema?

- **Hydrocortisone.** This is the doctor's treatment in its mildest form. Prescription steroid cream may be needed for more severe eczema.

- **Antihistamines**

- **Corticosteroids.** If other treatments fail, your doctor may prescribe oral corticosteroids..

- **Ultraviolet light therapy**. People with very severe eczema may benefit from therapy using ultraviolet light.

- **Immunosupressants**. Drugs that suppress the immune system may also be an option.

- **Immunomodulators**. This type of medicated cream helps treat eczema by controlling inflammation and reducing the immune system reactions.

- **Prescription-strength moisturizers.** These replace the barrier of the skin.

Some of these you now easily recognise as ways to calm down the allergies and also stop the system throwing up any immune problems. But what about hydrocortisone and corticosteroid creams, what are they about?

These are synthetic versions of the hormone secreted by the adrenals: cortisone. Long term use of them, acts in the same ways as long term stress does to our bodies. The adrenals become exhausted. This is such a well known phenomenon doctors have a checklist of things to watch for in children who have long term use of topical steroids. On that list is to watch for the risk of Cushing's Syndrome, a rare disorder where the pituitary gland instructs the adrenal to produce far too much cortisol. In addition to this, side effects of overuse of these very strong creams can also be growth defects. Those of you with a keen endocrine knowledge will know this also pertains to the pituitary.

In the Professional Stress Solution this adrenal exhaustion problem is addressed at length, as well as its relationship to the pituitary gland. Here, know that creams, over time, exhaust the adrenals. This then, must also be figured into your essential oil and vitamin choices on all accounts, but especially if they have been using steroids for any significant amount of time.

In the past it was also thought hydrocortisone thinned the skin. Whilst this can be so, recent research shows this is most likely to have happened to patients who have had their lesions covered with bandages, or can also happen with patients who have been using very strong topical creams over a prolonged period.

Now...that makes it seem like thinning is unlikely to happen, but...

The guidelines for prescription are not dissimilar to the way we would choose our creams. Use a moisturiser or lotion for wet and weeping eczema and an ointment base for thickened and hard skins.

It is also standard practice to mix two or more treatments, so a lotion for eczema on the face but an ointment for the more difficult to treat hands. Furthermore, for the hands and feet it is suggested that strong topical solutions should be used.

Where is it most likely you will find the skin getting ever more delicate? Yep, the hands. The eczema is sloughing off the skin too fast and over time the cream also is thinning it. Go back to The Dysfunction of the skin and you will be reminded of what problems of having a decreasing thickness of barrier cells will have.

Chapter 3 Eczema and Diet

Well, if you have made it thus far without plunging into despair of working out where to start, you deserve a medal. The food considerations for eczema bring their very own kind of brain strain. All I can say to you is reading it is harder than treating it. When you have a case history and a food diary in front of you it is simpler and clearer.

Food combinations

Ok, so here we are back to our house of cards, one solitary thing will tip the eczema over, but it won't always be the same thing. The problem with food intolerances (note the difference here, not allergies, these are far milder but enough to tip the house over) is they can be very slight.

In the *Essential Oil Liver Cleanse* I talk about how the toxicity of an organ makes it dysfunction. We talked in terms of percentages. If it is 30% toxic, an organ can only work to 70% power. 10% toxic and you have a better 90% power.

Intolerances work in a very similar way. They may be mild but if you stick enough of them on a sandwich together you will tip the house of cards over.

Example

I can't drink coffee at all now because it makes me feel stoned! It's a shame because I adore the smell. Earlier in my life though I was only slightly intolerant, so let's say I had 20% intolerance. I could drink it and have no problems at all.

Chocolate and I have a love hate relationship too. I love it, it hates me. We'll say 30%. Then let's add on a bit of red wine too... let's say 40%.

Right so on Monday, mostly I drank tea. No problems.

On Tuesday I met a friend in town and we had coffee and a slice of carrot cake. Nothing

On Wednesday, I went out to dinner, had roast beef with a red wine sauce, a glass of red, chocolate mousse and coffee after. The service was terrible and I ended up having an argument with my man because he made a comment that made me self conscious about my size.

Ouch, I just scratched so hard, I made myself bleed.

20% coffee + 30% chocolate+40% red wine= 90% toxicity from food intolerance.

Then I added a bit of anger on top too.

And the skin starts to flake away like a house of cards tumbling down....

The question is...which was the joker in the pack? All of them, but none of them on their own.

Can you see how it stacks up? It is ok to have a couple of weak spots in the house but one too many and it will go.

The key then, is to find ways to get rid of the weak spots.

We cleanse the liver of toxicity. (See Essential Oils Liver Cleanse) We address the personality and emotional issues which are causing the catalyst (See Professional Stress Solution). This might be through CBT, counselling, or maybe your oils alone will do the job. We check the back is straight and not nudging any nerves to send organic dysfunction. If you haven't already, download your chart of spinal misalignments from buildyourownreality.com/chiropractic.

We cleanse the digestive tracts and choose foods which will enable it to heal, and of course we heal the skin.

Let's look at possible nutritional defects first then we'll move onto food. If you have read my stress book, you will have some moments of déjà vu here, because I have simply copied some passages across. The roles of vitamin therapy don't change and my hands ache from typing! Again, a chart is available to help you at buildyourownreality.com/vitamins

Vitamin A – In its own right this does not contribute to eczema healing, however leaky gut will lose vitamin A resources and make it impossible to process zinc which is vital.

Vitamin B complex; B6, especially B12.

These vitamins contribute to the production of new skin cells and tissue. It also supports the nervous system, which is important for immunity and proper functioning health. Most importantly lowered vitamin B levels results in itchy and flaky skin. You may also recall it is the fuel for the liver. Without it our house of cards is going to topple.

Vitamin C – is a powerful antioxidant giving protection to skin damage. It is also necessary for vitamin B to absorb effectively.

Vitamin D - low levels have been proven to trigger itchiness. In all patients, you will find it useful to prescribe vitamin D

Vitamin E – Taking vitamin E reduces susceptibility to itching and dryness. It is a powerful antioxidant giving protection to skin damage too.

Magnesium

I'm going to get on my soapbox now in campaign for my beloved magnesium. A bit of background is, when I was carrying my last child I suffered a blood clot in my lungs. I was given a drug called Clexane which stripped all the calcium from my blood. No-one told me to take calcium supplements which I now know they should have done. This affected my already depleted levels of magnesium.

Some symptoms of depleted magnesium are:

Tics, muscle spasms and cramps restless legs, seizures, anxiety, and irregular heart rhythms migraine headaches, insomnia, depression, and chronic fatigue, amongst others. It can also be a source of problems for incontinence issues too. Many experts suspect magnesium may in fact be the key to Metabolic Syndrome.

The tell tale sign for me was my husband's biggest complaint in life. I am a massive fidget in bed. I have restless legs and as I am falling asleep, I jump very aggressively and suddenly. Then I read this was a classic sign of magnesium deficiency. I couldn't believe it! But yes, after just a few days of supplementing no more restless legs or jumping when I fall asleep. Not only that, no more PMT or migraines either.

What's more, when he was finally born, the child was a dreadful sleeper. I mean waking twenty or thirty times every night. The first night he slept through, he was aged four. A week earlier I started him on a children's supplement of magnesium. His concentration is better and his behaviour is very much improved. I deliberately left out an aspect of how a person becomes very yin. It is not likely to be genetically passed from mother to child, but it is definitely congenital. That is to say because my condition became so extreme when he was in utero, he was born the same way.

Magnesium people! It's the future!

And actually it makes sense because magnesium in fruit develops when it reaches maturity. What do we know about fruit retailing now? They pick food too early. Magnesium is naturally found in the largest quantities in leafy green vegetables, nuts, oily fish, fruit then whole grains. Strangely too, when you cook leafy greens, the magnesium efficiency increases too, same for grains and fruits.

How magnesium absorbs and is assimilated is important because people who experience large bouts of diarrhoea will not be able to assimilate it; the body's natural response is to expel it. So for people who are present with problems such as IBS or Crohns for instance you should administer in a different manner. Magnesium is better absorbed through the skin. Prescribe Epsom salts baths or magnesium chloride oil(which isn't actually an oil at all more a serum) for far better results.

The recommended daily allowance is 400mg per day so I prescribe 300 with the hope the rest will come from improved diet. Should we have misjudged and have prescribed too much then the body naturally dispels through diarrhoea

Calcium

You will notice from the chart on the pdf that calcium and magnesium sit on opposite lines. This is because they are wholly inter dependant on each other. You may remember from your chemistry lessons that elements are either positively or negatively charged. In the case of mg and Ca, they are both divalent cations translated as they both have a double positive charge. What this means is they compete for absorption in the body. The higher the level of calcium, the harder it is for the magnesium to absorb.

On the surface then, it looks like you should not supplement calcium. However between the ages of 30-35 a person loses the ability to store calcium and so after that age, yes it is advisable to do so. Since the calcium/ magnesium balance has a direct bearing on production of D3 aim for a supplement of this too.

Deficiency of D3 is thought to be a contributory factor in the development of many strains of cancer.

Copper

Every cell in the body requires copper, iron and zinc to function. I have therefore grouped these together. These are your most essential minerals.

Now the strange thing about copper is our bodies cannot manufacture or store it. Every bit of it either has to come from food or water intake. Any excess is excreted.

Copper's main jobs are to look after the brain, nervous system and cardiovascular system.

It contributes to:

- Brain development and the maintenance of brain health
- Effective communications between nerve cells
- Maintenance of healthy cells and connective tissue
- Wound healing
- The structural integrity of the cardiac muscles
- Growth of new blood cells

- Healthy immune response by contributing to the formation of white blood cells

Immediately, you should be able to see the connection between an inbalance in copper and how that might affect the skin.

Some foods are especially rich in copper. Most nuts (especially brazils and cashews), seeds (especially poppy and sunflower), chickpeas, liver and oysters are great sources. Whole food cereals, meat and fish generally contain sufficient copper to provide up to 50% of the required copper intake in a balanced diet.

In the UK we have the added advantage that our water runs through copper pipes and this helps a great deal. Put the water through a filter though and copper will be depleted along with many other elements.

Recommended daily intake is adults 1.2 mg and children 0.5-1 mg

Zinc

Stress decreases zinc which in turn causes copper levels to rise. Zinc is actually responsible for over a 100 different processes in the body but again edited highlights. It has a calming effect on the brain. If you have an upsurge in copper, mood cannot be stabilised. Low zinc is found in patients with depression, most notably those with post natal depression.

Again this is a vital component to wound healing. The largest threat to an eczema suffer is that zinc fails to absorb correctly because of cell permeability and a leaky gut. Mal-absorption can also be established because of a deficiency in vitamins A & D.

Iron

Again, the body cannot manufacture iron. It must be brought into the body via food. I'm sure most of you will remember the functions of iron from your lessons on the circulatory system, but for those of you who were not listening at the back...

It is vital for:

- The production of red blood cells
- Transportation of haemoglobin around the body
- It binds to carbon dioxide to bring about the exchange of gases
- It aids the conversion of sugar into energy
- It is a building block for the production of enzymes, amino acids, hormones and neuro transmitters

- It supports the immune system

Iron is found in good supply in:

Liver, meat, beans, nuts, dried fruit, such as dried apricots, whole grains, such as brown rice, fortified breakfast cereals, soybean flour, most dark-green leafy vegetables, such as watercress and curly kale. Although it is a great source of iron, liver should be avoided in pregnancy because of its high levels of vitamin A

Choline

Although usually classified as a B vitamin because it has very similar traits and often works in conjunction with B, choline is recognised as an essential nutrient. Initially it was found in the pancreas. This was an exciting discovery because choline stops the liver accumulating fat. The excitement rose to fever pitch when scientists were able to establish choline is present in every cell in the human body.

Its job is to transmit lipids to ensure the liver holds onto harmful fats and cholesterols and then provokes it to produce good cholesterol. It is also an important component of lecithin which is necessary for effective liver function. Its high levels of anti-oxidants support development, healing and preservation of organs and glands and essential to the health of liver, bladder and kidneys.

Most importantly for eczema suffers is it is involved in nerve processing and plays a part in balancing mood and sleep as well as memory.

Naturally, the body can synthesize choline itself, but most of the resources come from beef, cod fish, salmon, prawns, eggs, milk, peanuts, wheat germ and vegetables.

The recommended daily allowance of choline is 425-550mg daily.

Biotin

This is involved in the metabolism of fats, proteins and carbohydrates and so therefore the production of energy. Sometimes you might see this listed as Vitamin H.

It is naturally found in milk, liver, egg yolks, yeast and dried peas.

Deficiency of biotin is rare, but can be provoked by eating of rare egg whites. Whites contain high levels of avidin, a compound which binds biotin and prevents it from performing. Cooking egg whites reduces this binding process. At first glance you might wonder at the people who gulp raw eggs from the glass but also meringues, royal icing and mayonnaise all contain raw eggs.

Determine Food Allergies

Even without identifying food allergies, avoiding all wheat and dairy products such as milk, cheese, etc. will be helpful, since most people have allergies to these.

Eating alkaline foods helps eczema a great deal. Green leafy vegetable and fresh fruit, are alkaline. Other alkaline foods include: Asparagus, Onions, Vegetable Juices, Parsley, Raw Spinach, Broccoli, Garlic, Lemons, Watermelon, Limes, Dates, Figs, Melons, Grapes, Papaya, Kiwi, Berries, Apples, Pears, Raisins, Olive Oil, Lemon Water, etc.

Acid-forming foods will usually increase symptoms.

Avoid: processed food, junk food, refined carbohydrates like white bread, white rice, white sugar, etc, soda, alcohol, coffee, tea, dairy, pizza, candy, cookies, eggs, peanuts, gelatin, meat, fish, chocolate.

Officially, raw food works best for treating eczema, followed by steamed and boiled. If however your patient seems to be in a very weakened state, or has been under stress for a length of time, I would suggest putting them on a high protein intake of white meats for a fortnight to give their amino acid production a kick start. This is detailed more fully in the Professional Stress Solution. **Avoid microwaved, fried, and baked foods as much as possible.**

Avoid excessive amounts of citrus and sour items. These can make itching worse.

Hydration is very important. Not only will it add moisture to the skin cells but it helps to flush out toxins from the body that aggravate symptoms.

Work **essential fatty acids** such as **flax, flax seed oil, extra virgin olive** and **coconut oil** into their diet.

For infants, delaying solid foods may be helpful for symptoms, if there is a family history of allergies, hay fever, asthma, food allergies.

Juice therapy with **black currants, red grapes, carrot, beet, spinach, cucumber, parsley, green juice, wheat grass** is a great boost for the system too

Right from the beginning of the treatment I would recommend you try to encourage your patient to write a detailed food diary. Sheer mental application, when it is done this way can usually help you to pin point protagonists but allergy testing works very well too.

Two other disciplines I find very useful are medical dowsing and kinesiology. I am a qualified medical dowser, but not kinesiologist. I can let you have some basic hints on what this involves, so you can decide if you wanted to take your skills further.

Dowsing works on the same principle as water divining. It reads a vibration and then it answers a question yes or no. Is there water there? Does this person need?

My late step father was the genius of all geniuses at this, and if you search the name Michael Cook you can see him in action. He was the only person James Randy was unable to disprove in all the years of his paranormal shows. In the programme Mike dowses a map to find an object, but the process is exactly the same. Near the end of his life he was the Chairman of the British Society of Dowsers.

I use the same process as him, because he taught me, but there is no set way of doing this. You need a pendulum of some description. I use a pointy crystal because it is easy to see what direction it points to on lists. I have seen him do it with a bathroom plug!

I have a list of vitamins and minerals and I simply go down the list checking yes they need it, no they don't.

To start to dowse, the most important thing is to tell yourself you can do it. Then ask a question you know the answer to. I use: Am I a girl? Then, Am I a boy? That way I can see how the pendulum swings for yes and how it goes for no. Usually, but not always you have a circle for no, and it will swing in a straight line for yes.

That's all there is to it, but I have to say I do mistrust it enough to look back at the list and want to see valid reasons for the choices. Naturally this doesn't stop at vitamins and minerals, you can discern essential oils, crystals, chakras...the list is endless really. If there are some bizarre choices that come up, personally I miss them out, but actually that probably defeats the process.

Kinesiology is the most fun you can have without having cake! This really is an applied science, and specialist training is required but....

Did you know your body has no resistance to any element it is deficient in?

The idea is to hold the element in one and hold the other arm out to your side at shoulder height. Now get someone to push your raised arm down. If you have adequate resources of the element in your body, you will be able to hold your arm high. If you are deficient, no matter how hard you try to maintain that muscle composure, you won't be able to. It is really funny the first time you experience it, because you really cannot hold your arm up. Get someone to have a play with the oils in your box, or if you want a real giggle go and annoy a sales assistant by doing it in the health food store with the vitamins. Again, I have to say, you are not qualified, therefore not insured so write your list of muscle killers and then go and check the text books before you get prescribing.

Subtle Energies

Ok so we have covered the science, until our brains feel like Bunsen burners now I think. Let's have a very quick look at the metaphysical side. You are all, I hope familiar with the expression the holistic approach. We are made up of three entities acting as one; the mind, the body and a spiritual aspect too.

This book has I hope shown you specific ways the emotions affect the way our physical body functions. Certainly too, it reflects how a person feel about the situation they find themselves in, in their lives generally. What's more, should the spirit decide you are not living your life in the way you should, it will definitely through you a health curb ball.

But how does this emanate from being this internal/internal unquantifiable thing...the spirit...to being a skin condition?

This is covered far more deeply in *The Mind Body Spirit of Essential Oils*, but....

The aura is the seat of the spirit. It has seven layers and it acts as both a barometer of feelings and emotions but also for health. The chakras are wheels of energy which emanate though the aura, then through the physical body, passing through the spine. These chakras vitalise the physical body, but emotions can jar them open or closed preventing them from working effectively. Without this energy, the organs lose energy and start to dysfunction. The most likely chakra to be dysfunctional, specifically for eczema, is the solar plexus chakra, and to come extent the sacral too.

There is a chart for you to use in your treatments at: buildyourownreality.com/chakra-chart

Chiropractic

The spine plays an important part in health. In fact I should rephrase that. It plays an absolutely vital part in health. If vertebrae are misaligned they can tilt and run on nerves. These are known in chiropractic as subluxions. These subluxions cause organic dysfunction.

There is a chart available to help you with this section at: buildyourownreality.com/chiropractic.

What I will say is with eczema, the causes are so diverse it can almost be useful sending them to a chiropractor anyway. The chakras also run through the spine and the aura, so if there are misalignments, you also have this breakdown between the spirit and the physical body too. Again, you can expect this to radiate into dis-ease of some description.

In the chart, you will see C3 and T11 are most likely to be your main protagonists but, that is certainly not the entire story. If you are not sure how to check for misalignments of the spine, here is a quick over view for you.

At the very least, the shoulder mantle and the hip bones should be parallel. Misalignments in the back will tip them, but also every day activities such as carrying heavy shopping or shoulder bags will do it too. It is a useful exercise to do this exercise yourself in front of the mirror to see if you can see any possible issues on your own body too.

The best course of action is to assess this just in the underwear. Use your thumbs to isolate the top edge of your hips. Have a look in the mirror. Do they look level with each other? Now also look at the line of your shoulders? Does that look right too?

Problems with the spine try to correct themselves by over compensating. If your left hip seems higher, it is usual see the right shoulder is raised to try and balance it out. This can give the spine a rather disconcerting letter S appearance. In the same way if it hasn't "corrected" itself, you will see the right hip, right shoulder-up interplay. Neither is the correct stance. Correct is parallel.

Does the pelvis look like it is vertically straight too? In particular child birth can cause the iliac joints to rotate or even separate the front of the pelvis too. You can see this as if someone walks a bit like a duck sticking her tail out (pelvis pushed back), or the wild west cowboy sticking his bits forward as he walks (and pelvis pushed forward or, in fact, under).

Checking for specific vertebrae misalignments is easier to do on someone else. To the untrained hand small subluxtions are more difficult to discern. Listen to your hands and trust your instincts. Even if the naked eye can't see it, your fingers will probably pick it up. Remember even a very tiny misalignment can be extremely detrimental to health.

A great time to check for misalignments is during your back massage. Before you sart to massage, it is good practice to check the lie of the feet. Ask your patient to lie on their back. Lift a foot in either hand and let them gently drop to the couch. You are looking to see how they naturally fall when the patient has their hips square on the bed. They should fall to the bed and then flop open, hells together-ish and toes pointing outwards. Imagine where the clock hands are at ten to two. This is correct alignment. Also just check...is one leg sitting longer than the other? It's amazing how many times you can miss that clue if you are not looking.

Regardless of the school of massage you have been taught, most back massages include a section when you rake gently down the spine. This action is perfect for checking spinal position. To discern any misalignments use your index and middle fingers. Place one either side of the spine. Gently trace down and be attentive to the positions of the bones. I usually do three passes at this, a) because it feels so relaxing to the patient b) I am looking to double check my findings all of the time. In order to really listen to my hands and not be swayed by what I can/can't see, I tend to do this with my eyes closed and let instinct take over. I will however, at this point say, it is unusual for me to do a massage on an eczema patient. Once you have the idea though you will find it easier to check the patient whist they are standing up, or alternatively just get them to jump on the couch for you.

It may be obvious to say there might be, and probably is, more than one bone out of place. This can feel like a red herring when you begin to look, especially if they are next to each other. This can happen, and indeed it is even more important to get your patient care if you discern this. Two vertebrae, close together, are referred to as a motion segment; these put extra pressure on the disc causing it to deteriorate over time.

I can't stress how important it is to get the spine straight. You can do months and months of essential oil therapy only to find this could have been the root of the problem all of the time. What I will say is it is not a "one session, you're cured" system, I'm afraid. The muscles holding your spine in place get to quite like where they sit and whilst the manipulation itself does not hurt, the muscles ache the next day. Actually you can feel like you have been under a steam roller!!! The muscular tissue will fight the process all of the way, especially the muscles which now need to stretch more to accommodate the vertebra's new position. In the meantime, every time a muscle contracts back into relaxation, it will try to bring the spine with it.

Think of it a bit like doing the splits. Every day, there is a bit more stretch. The same applies to manipulation. The process takes as long as it takes, but 3-5 sessions can be a good pointer as to how long "training" will take. I will stress again, chiropractic doesn't hurt. The muscles do ache, but for the most part, people feel better, freer, looser, after a manipulation, but not worse. Many people then decide to go on to have regular treatments, a bit like having the car serviced, to keep them tuned up.

Cranial manipulation can give you a headache for a couple of days though, I have to say. Although less likely to apply with an eczema patient, since there are links with migraine, this might be useful for you to know.

Manipulation can unlock emotions in the same way as I am sure you have seen massage do. Of particular note here is work done on the coccyx and sacro-iliac joints. Whilst you should be able to rely on your chiropractor to prepare your patient (or explain it, if it arises, depending on his approach), from a professional point of view it is worth knowing weepiness, fatigue, feelings of vulnerability and general sensitivity are not uncommon after work has been done on these areas. That being said, my husband has been having regular chiropractic treatments for nigh on twenty years and I have never seen evidence of this with him so it is certainly not a given.

Your patient is at an advantage, having your treatments at the same time, of course. Your massage pummels and loosens the muscles making them suppler and more receptive to manipulation. This helps the process. A good add on treatment for you to offer is a blend to get rid of the muscle waste after the process. A bit of juniper is very effective for shifting the lactic acid build up and of course lavender and camomile give them some respite from the aches and pains too.

The Meridians

Running up and down the body too, are pathways of energy called meridians. You will see these on the pdf. If the energy becomes blocked in some way, disease arises. We unblock these channels by using acupressure points to allow qi to flow more effectively.

Incidentally, acupoints are a wonderful way of releasing emotional blockages from the organs too.

Acupressure for eczema

So far, traditional medicine refuses to accept aromatherapy might be able to help eczema, although they will concede it has psychological benefits which lead to healing. Traditional Chinese Medicine though, that's another story. Acupressure has lots of converts and evidence to back it up. On particular trial used just one point LI11 on atopic dermatitis patients over a period of four weeks and saw significant changes in both the itching and the lichenification of the skin. Another trial showed the same point helped to alleviate chemically induced dermatitis in rats. A third study used (bilateral BL13, and unilateral LI11, ST36, SP10, SP6) to successfully treat the poor rodents, who had this time been irritated with capsicum. Yet another set of ratties, with AD this time, were treated with pharmacopuncture (Injecting Chinese herbs into the points) into BL3, and were seen to have improvements

A set of 30 *human* volunteers with AD were aggravated with an allergen and were then treated with LI11 and SP10 which showed significant reduction in the itching and hyper-sensitivity as fast as 10 minutes after treatment

Acupressure will help the body to eliminate the toxin and it will also give the patients organs a kick start to get them going.

To recap the list is:

LI11, ST36, SP10, SP6 BL3, bilateral BL13

These are shown on your chart available from buildyourownreality.com/eczema-points

Build them into your massage or show the patient how to stimulate them daily. I tend to use ones on the legs and hands if I can, so it is easy for them to reach tem without being a contortionist.

Remember these are strong healers in their own right. Then you are adding essential oils to them. DO NOT OVER STIMULATE. 30 seconds pressure each day is ample.

If you have never used acupressure points before, it is worth finding a couple on yourself to see how they feel. Can you feel tension in your temples? What about just under your eyebrows? These are sinus points. A good migraine one is in the flap of your skin between the thumb and your first finger. There are some which often feel tender at the base of the back of your skull. My points just under my ears on the end of the jaw are often painful too.

Apply pressure to the point. If it feels painful it is blocked. Firm, but not hard fingertip pressure will empty the blockage. If it is a fold of skin, like on the hand, or on the ears, pinching works well too.

Now I use these meridians as sites to place essential oils. Where do you place oils to cleanse the liver, for instance? The liver is inside. Rubbing the oils along the hepatic meridian speeds detoxification.

Essential oil therapy

So we are here....the bit you have been waiting for. I hope you haven't found it too long winded. I do love a bit of physiology can you tell? I do think it is important though, because if you can talk science and facts, and data and really understand it...well then you can sell it. Fundamentally that's what I want you take away from this book. I want you to be able to say to your client "I think I can help, because think this might be what is happening to you. These are the oils I will use, and these are the reasons why."

A couple of disclaimers:

For the purists amongst you, not all of these are essential oils. Some are absolutes too.

Also, whilst I have tried to match the oils up with scientific evidence, some I could not do. This does not mean they are not correctly listed. It means an appropriate trial has not yet taken place. If there is negative advice, I have listed that too.

Massage

To massage or not to massage: that is the question.

Firstly, I should say if a person has bad eczema I tend not to think massage is your best treatment avenue because a) it is contraindicated over broken skin but mainly b) I think they might be embarrassed. Certainly offer it, but in my opinion creams and lotions work far better.

A well published clinical trial under taken by the School of Applied Science, London demonstrated that whilst massage on childhood eczema had very short term effect, in the long term, the essential oils actually exacerbated the eczema. In a moment, I'll explain why I think this is relevant. The most popular choices of oils by the mothers of the children were: sweet marjoram, frankincense, German chamomile, myrrh, thyme, benzoin, spike lavender and Litsea cubeba. What they did determine though, was the positive effects of touch the massage was having on the children.

So then, possibly not massage with essential oils, but stroking in a lotion most definitely has benefits.

Bases

As I said earlier choose your base according to the condition of the eczema. If it is wet and weeping, use a lotion. An ointment works better for toughened skin. It is good for knees, elbows etc.

Research by Nottingham University shows the most effective treatment by far, is moisturising with an emollient base. Be absolutely sure your base is water based, not oil based which could confuse sebaceous glands into under producing and causing drier skin.

If you'd like to see Michael Cork, Head of Academic Dermatology at the University of Sheffield speaking about why this is important, (He's the guy I cited describing how eczema affects the iron rods in the skin cells) there is a short video here: https://www.youtube.com/watch?v=1RDtPIWfF9c . It is a very useful guide.

Baths

Oatmeal and wheat germ baths work well, as do Epsom salts. Ensure your patient knows not to use soaps because they are too harsh.

Showers

Not so much a base here, as a comment. It is useful to have a water filter fitted to the shower to reduce sensitivity

Carrier Oils

We are straight into the world of controversy now. In the 1990s Evening Primrose gained a medicinal license for its treatment of eczema based on its high levels of Gamma Linolenic Acid. Early trials had shown good effects on skin, but very quickly the medical profession turned tail, decided it didn't work and revoked its license.

There are pages and pages on the internet citing EPO as not working. Actually the clinical trials were for orally ingested EPO, not oil. Indeed in 2008, a study in India directly opposed this, saying it did indeed improve eczema in their subjects. Again though, this was a trial taking oral capsules.

Borage oil too, had a bit of a hey-day, because that has even higher levels of GLA. Again trials with oral capsules have not shown improvement in symptoms. With borage though, we have a bit more to go on. Firstly, the medics say it a good choice for babies with nappy rash, known to be a close cousin of eczema. But, excitingly a 2007 study of 32 young children with atopic dermatitis were asked to wear undershirts coated with borage oil for two weeks. The sixteen children with the placebo showed no improvement, but all sixteen children who had worn the borage showed significant improvement. Water loss from their skin was radically reduced.

Calendula is also high on the list. This will not come as a surprise to anyone since this plant has been used for nappy rash since time immemorial. However in 1996, trials showed it to be by far the most effective treatment for dermatitis caused by radiation in breast cancer patients.

Atopic Eczema – Borage Oil

                Evening Primrose Oil

Contact Dermatitis – Calendula Oil

Essential Oils

The doctors agree the most effective treatment they have for eczema is a patented cream made from Chamomile, Kamillosan®. In clinical trials this performs *slightly* better than hydrocortisone. This is made from Roman Chamomile. Be aware not to use matricaria as this is proven to cause sensitisation in some patients.

Research in Ethiopia into more economical ways to treat patients with eczema showed incredible results. Using a cream with 3% dilution of anti-fungal thyme mixed with a 10% Chamomile, 66% of patients were cleared of their eczema completely, compared with 28.5% of the placebo group, who were treated with a blank moisturising base.

To stop itching

Lavender – *Lavendula angustifolia* only in small doses as it will dry the skin further.

Camomile – *Anthemis nobilis*

Valerian – *Valeriana officianalis*

A 2002 study in Japan examined the effects of inhaling valerian on patients with AD. They found not only did the mood of the patients improve but also the skin scaliness and redness. Whilst the paper recommends inhalation, I would also advocate mild dilution in the cream to help with itching, but also sleep.

To treat the surface eczema
Geranium, Calendula

I understand people with red hair have a higher sensitivity rate to geranium. I don't know why this might be. Check for sensitivity first. So far I have not come across anyone who is allergic to both geranium and marigold.

Geranium – Pelargonium graveolens

On the surface there is no reason for this oil to work, but I have seen it do incredible things for eczema. So far, I have not been able to isolate any clinical evidence to support this claim...

However, it regulates the adrenal hormones, it works as an interface between the emotions and the mental facilities and also, maybe fundamentally, this year has been proven to be extremely effective in eradicating *candida albacans* in clinical trials.

Calendula – Calendula officinalis

The benefits of using calendula carrier and essential oil are myriad. You might find an old article I wrote about calendula useful here buildyourownreality.com/calendula

To heal broken skin

Myrrh – Communis myrrha

The ultimate skin healer, in my opinion.

Galbanum – *Ferula Galbaniflua*

Particularly if it is ulcerated.

Benzoin – *Styrax benzoin*

In the National Library of Medicine, there are no less than 21 papers citing dermatitis break outs after use of benzoin tincture in dressings after surgery (It seems popular in nose jobs for some reason!). We can draw two questionable conclusions here: Firstly it seems to be seen as quite a reputable post operative medication 2) It seems interesting to me the paper which slates massage for children with AD makes no mention of mixes being used *without* benzoin. Does that mean then, other oils have been simply rejected as useless, when there are two oils which are questionable in the mix. German Chamomile, definitely is a sensitizer, and now this....

That being said....it wouldn't put me off using benzoin once I tested for skin sensitivity. It is a wonderful skin healer. I'd be the first to jump to its defence. It seems I'm not the only one. A paper written by the Contact Dermatitis Clinic at the Skin Cancer Foundation, wanted to know what had happened to poor old benzoin too.

They say in their report this year, there have been less than 30 cases of contact dermatitis ever recorded against benzoin, and none in the last decade. But in their trial of 477 people, 45 had reactions. 14 had strong reactions, but of these 11 had also had a cross reaction with either a fragrance mix, balsam of peru, colophony (rosin for violin bows or ballet pointes amongst other uses) or tea tree.

So then, use it, but use it carefully; not least because by the nature of the treatment these are people who have allergens and sensitivities. Above all, watch what you are blending it with.

To reduce scarring

Jasmine – *Jasminum officianale*

Anti allergenic

Lemon Balm – *Melissa officinalis*

Circulation for varicose eczema

Geranium – *Pelargonium graveolens*

To cleanse the liver

More in the liver book, but for general purposes

Hepatic oils

Chamomile - *Camomile maroc*

Eucalyptus- *Eucalyptus globulus*

Fatty Liver

Ginger – *Zingiber officinale* – Ginger is showing positive early signs of eradicating fatty liver in rats.

To cleanse heavy metal debris

Oakmoss resin – *Evernia prunastri*

Oakmoss again is an oil with a chequered history. Once the darling of perfumery, it was found to be a sensitising agent. Legislation in January 2010 restricted its usage to 0.1% dilution.

Just as an aside, because it is interesting about what happens to essential oils, and nothing at all to do with eczema...Guerlain, who had two chypre perfumes which were heavy in Oakmoss, decided there was no way they could possibly operate without them. Their perfumer Thierry Wasser, created a molecule without 100ppm atranol and chloroatranol, the two sensitising components.

Benzoin – *Styrax benzoin*

The adrenals

Again see the Professional Stress Solution

Mandarin =*Citrus reticulata*

Digestive cleansers

Cardamom- *Elattaria cardamomum*

Ginger –*Zingiber officinalis*

Kidneys

Chamomile - *Camomile Maroc*

Frankincense – *Boswellia carterii*

Geranium – *Pelargonium graveolens*

Jasmine – *Jasminum officianale*

Gall bladder

Celery Seed –*Apium graveolens*

I like this one because it works on the liver and gall bladder together

Helichrysm - *Helichrysum italicum*

This is a general tonic, but also cleans the blood.

Spleen

Helichrysm - *Helichrysum italicum*

Geranium – *Pelargonium graveolens*

Parasites

Digestive system

Lime - *Citrus aurantifolia*

Oregano - *Origanum vulgare*

Lemon verbena - *Aloysia citrodora*

Pine - *Pinus sylvestris*

Blood

Lime - *Citrus aurantifolia*

Garlic - *Allium sativum*

Lemon grass - *Cymbopygon nardus*

Tissues

Lime - *Citrus aurantifolia*

Cypress - *Cupressus semperivens*

Vermifuge

Tea tree - *Maleleuca alternifolia*

Thyme - *Thymus vulgaris*

Excreted toxins

Birch (white) - *Betula alba*

Insect bites

From Europe, US and Australia

Eucalyptus - *Eucalyptus globulus*

From Africa

Calendula - *Calendula officinalis*

From Asia

Anise - *Pimpinella anisum*

From Food

Violet leaf - *Viola odorata*

Thyme - *Thymus vulgaris*

Candida albacans & Malessezzia furfur

A study by the University of Poland has confirmed the following oils "exhibit significant activity reducing the presence/quantity of important C. albicans virulence factors."

Geranium - *Pelargonium graveolens*

Citronella - *Cymbopygon nardus*

Lemon Balm - *Melissa officinalis*

Clove - *Syzygium aromaticum*

Other anti-fungal oils worth considering are:

Lavender, myrrh, tea tree, thyme, lemon

Geopathic stress
Birch – *Betula alba*

Disinfects the aura of VDU positive ions

Oils for the emotions
Amber – (No Latin name as actually it is a fossilised resin, not a plant)

Lifts trauma

Benzoin –*Styrax benzoin*

Helps a person break free from mental fetters and physical hold ups

Calendula – *Calendula officinalis*

Helps a person see the complexity of an issue, in this case their house of cards

Chamomile- *Camomile Maroc*

Calms the mind and relieves stress

Cedarwood Atlas –*Cedrus atlantica*

Clears unwanted thoughts

Frankincense – *Boswellia Carterii*

Instils courage and confidence

Helichrysm – *Helichrysm italicum*

Help the sufferer be strong and prevents them from being weighed down by the eczema

Myrrh –*Communis myrrha*

Calms the nervous system

Parsley Leaf- *Petroselenium crispum*

Nervous relationships with parents

Homeopathic dose 1/15th drop (see Complete Guide to Clinical Aromatherapy and Essential Oils for The Physical Body)

Rose Otto – *Rosa damascena*

Brings about a stillness of the brain

Oils for the chakras

Skin disorders tend, most often, to show themselves in the crown chakra, but I think the solar plexus and chakra would certainly come into play if emotions seem to be the issue here. Likewise, watch how the throat chakra changes through the treatments as they begin to address how they express themselves.

Crown

Angelica - *Angelica archangelica*

Citronella – *Cymbopogon nardus*

Frankincense - *Boswellia carterii*

Palma Rosa - *Cympobogon martinii*

Hyacinth - *Hyacinthus orientalis*

Cumin - *Cuminum cuminum*

Violet Leaf - *Viola odorata*

Sandalwood - *Santalum album*

Lemon - *Citrus limonum*

Juniper - *Juniperus communis*

Pineal

Anise – *Pimpinella anisum*

Lavender French *Lavandula stoechas*

Lemon – *Citrus limonum*

Lemongrass – *Cymbopogon citratus*

Birch – *Betula alba*

Camomile Roman *Anthemis nobilis*

Cardomon - *Elettaria cardamomum*

Clary Sage - *Salvia sclarea*

Hop - *Humulus lupulus*

Myrrh – *Communis myrrha*

Throat

Cade, *Juniperus oxycedrus*

Cajuput - *Melaleuca leucadendra*

CedarwoodAtlas - *Cedrus atlantica*

Cypress - *Cupressus semperivens*

Dill - *Anethum graveolens*

Garlic – *Allium sativum*

Ginger – *Zingiber officinale*

Grapefruit – *Citrus paridisii*

Helichrysm - *Helichrysum italicum*

Oregano – *Origanum vulgare*

Rosemary – *Rosmarinus officinalis*

Bulgarian Lavender – *Lavendula angustifolia*

Rose Otto – *Rosa damascena*

Peppermint – *Mentha piperita*

Neroli – *Citrus aurantium*

Heart

Amber (No botanical name)

Basil - *Ocimum basilicum*

Bay, *Pimenta Racemosa*

Benzoin *Styrax benzoin*

Calendula-*Calendula officinalis*

Caraway - *Carum carvi*

English Lavender – Lavendula angustifolia

Galbanum - *Ferula galbaniflua*

Lavandin – *Lavendula x intermedia*

Mandarin - *Citrus reticulata*

Mimosa - *Acacia Dealbata*

Myrtle - *Myrtus Communis*

Ginger - *Zingiber officinale*

Orange - *Citrus Cinensis*

Parsley Seed - *Petroselinium sativum*

Sage - *Salvia officinalis*

Spearmint - *Mentha spicata*

Sweet Fennel - *Foeniculum vulgare*

Tangerine - *Citrus reticulata Blanco var*

Thyme - *Thymus vulgare*

Vanilla - *Vanilla planifolia*

Vertivert - *Vetyveria zizanoides*

Rose Maroc - *Rosa damascena*

Rose geranium - *Pelargonium Rosa*

Lime - *Citrus aurantifolia*

Solar plexus

Cade - *Juniperus oxycedrus*

Cajuput - *Melaleuca leucadendra*

Cedarwood Atlas - *Cedrus Atlantica*

Cypress – *Cupressus semperivens*

Dill - *Anethum Graveolens*

Garlic – *Allium sativum*

Ginger - *Zingiber officinale*

Grapefruit - *Citrus paradisii*

Helichrysm - *Helichrysm italicum*

Oregano - *Origanum vulgare*

Rosemary - *Rosmarinus officinale*

Bulgarian Lavender - *Lavendula angustifolia*

Rose Otto - *Rosa damascena*

Peppermint - *Mentha piperita*

Neroli - *Citrus auriantum*

Sacral

Black Pepper - *Piper nigrum*

Bulgarian Lavender – *Lavendula angustifolia*

Celery Seed, *Apium Graveolens*

Cinnamon Bark - *Cinnamomum Zeylanicum*

Coriander - *Coriandrum Sativum*

Neroli - *Citrus aurantium*

Niaouli – *Maleleuca quinquenervia*

Pimento Berry – *Pimenta officinalis*

Rose de Mai – *Rosa centifolia*

Rosewood - *Aniba Rosaeodora*

Ylang Ylang - *Cananga odorata*

Tonka Bean - *Dipteryx odorata*

Peppermint – *Mentha piperita*

Rose Otto - *Rosa damascena*

Root

Clove - *Syzygium aromaticum*

Benzoin – *Styrax benzoin*

Oakmoss – *Evernia prunastri*

Patchouli – *Pogostemon patchouli*

Spikenard - *Nardostachys jatamansi*

Vetiver - *Vetyveria zizanoides*

Conclusion

Well as the rabbit said with a carrot in his mouth, "That's all Folks!"

It seems appropriate too, since carrots are hepatic!

It's a minefield isn't it? But I hope you have enjoyed the adventure, and have my fingers crossed your own house of cards is still standing and I haven't completely knocked you over with all the information. If you haven't already, make sure you download your charts. After all it was included in the price of the book, so you've already paid for it. Best get your money's worth!

There is no doubt eczema is a horrible illness. Personally I can't imagine anything worse than hearing your child screaming from the agony of it. In your hands, at this moment, you have life changing information. Acupressure points which will stop itching in mere moments, vitamins again proven to reduce the itching and essential oils to treat every facet of the illness. With eczema though, you are never treating just one patient. The wife whose husband won't go to the beach because he'll have to take his shirt off, the mum who cries herself to sleep in exhaustion after another hellish day scared for her child, the father who proudly watches his son leave for university confident his skin won't let him down...all of these will thank you too.

Now you are armed with every possible piece of data you need to gain clients, I would urge you to also read Sales Strategies for Gentle Souls. This in depth healing knowledge coupled with in depth sales training will super charge your business. I promise you, your bank manager won't know what's hit him. There is only one downside to this ferocious combination; it'll make the tax man grin too!

I am sure by now, you have grasped there are other books in the series, I hope you'll feel you want to get a couple more in the future. It means I'm doing my job right! I'd love it too, if you would please take the time to post me a review. These really make a difference in helping me to sell more books, but it's nice to hear what you thought too.

You know what I'd love to read on there? What was the most useful thing you will take away from the book? It's a great way for others to check they haven't missed anything vital too.

Speak soon I hope, and successful healing

Review and buy!

Bye!

Liz

Other works by the author

Book 1 - The Complete Guide to

Clinical Aromatherapy & Essential Oils for the Physical Body

Essentially...essential oils for beginners, talented novices and intermediate aromatherapists

Let me ask you, why do you want a book on aromatherapy?

Do you want to learn how to care for your family naturally?

Perhaps you have a franchise selling essential oils and want to know more about what they can do?

Maybe you love the delicious scents and want understand how these beautiful things come to heal.

I wonder if you have started to learn and now want to discover how to build on your knowledge.

Whatever you are looking for this book has something for you.

- Details of how to treat over 60 conditions with essential oils
- Profiles of over 100 natural plant essences and their safety data

- Descriptions of 15 carrier oils and their applications not only for massage but also adding to creams and lotions.
- Comprehensive data of how the chemistry of an oil will affect its actions
- In depth insights into how professional aromatherapists blend...including their 13 favourite recipes from their practices.

Including....

- Sensuous aromatherapy blends by a qualified sex therapist
- Two blends for labour by the midwife running an aromatherapy program on an NHS maternity ward
- A blend for depression by a qualified mental health

PLUS....

10 bonus essential oil monographs and a complementary hypnotherapy relaxation download.

Discount vouchers of treatments courses and products by participating therapists.

AND.... for those of you who would like to contribute, there is a chance to make a donation to cancer research too.

This is my gift to you.

FREE - From 30.11.14

Book 2 Essential Oils for Mind Body Spirit

The Holistic Medicine of Clinical Aromatherapy

Healing the skin, easing the tummy ache or getting someone to sleep is easy with essential oils. Anyone can do it. The joy of healing, though, comes from peeling back the layers of the disease, almost like a detective to find out exactly what caused it in the first place.

Consider this book to be lesson 2 in The Secret Healer Series.

You have mastered which oil to use for what and why...this book takes you step by step though the ancient healing mechanisms of the aura, the chakras and meridians but also explores how that ties in with the latest scientific discoveries into how the emotions affect our health. Using Candace Pert's remarkable "Molecules of Emotion" research, The Secret Healer shows you *where* to look for healing links and *why*.

- Uncover how a certain recurrent negative emotion can be the trigger to make you ill?
- Understand internal processes that mean that psychology, neurology and immunology are quintessentially, and inextricably linked.

- Learn how to use essential oils control your emotions and in turn bring about a far greater standard of wellness.
- Discover mindblowing research that shows the emotions we experience are actually the sensations of neuropeptides triggering our organs to do their jobs
- Reflect on the wonder of Chinese medicine and ancient healing being completely accurate in their healing mechanisms for thousands of years…now that science proves it to be so.

Essential Oils for The Mind Body Spirit couples ancient wisdom with cutting edge science. This is the knowledge the drug companies hope you never find out and our doctors pray we all will.

A short write up, for a book that will change your life. I promise you, when you read the latest findings of psychoimmunolgy, you will never waster another day on being angry again.

Book 3 The Essential Oil Liver Cleanse

The Professional Aromatherapist's Liver Detox

We are warned of the threats of heart attacks, strokes and cancer, especially if we are overweight.

What is kept quieter is doctors have established a link between toxicity in the liver and metabolic syndrome, the condition that leads to many of these conditions. What's more non fatty liver disease is known to underlie many other conditions such as ezcema, allergies and headaches.

The scandal is just how many of our livers are struggling under the strain of over processed foods, pharmaceutical debris and actually even our own bad tempers!

This book explains:

- The importance of the liver and its functions
- How it becomes dysfunctional and how to interpret warning signposts
- How to cleanse and nourish using not just essential oils, but also vitamins and minerals and diet.
- The strange correlation between how our emotions translate negativity into disease.
- How to implement other therapies such as chiropractic, acupressure and counselling and how to secure fantastic referrals.

This book is best used in tandem with The Professional Stress Solution to benefit from the complementary healing. Use Sales Strategies for Gentle Souls to create a marketing plan to use your new found knowledge to smash your competition out of the water!!!

Book 4 The Professional Stress Solution

Essential Oils and Holistic Health Stress Management Techniques for The Professional Aromatherapist

Stress is pandemic in our society.

Scientists agree it plays a quintessential role in how likely it is we will suffer from chronic and possibly fatal illnesses in the future. Risk factors of metabolic syndrome, diabetes, stroke and heart disease are increased through stress.

The daft thing is....aromatherapy can do amazing things to ease it, and potentially aromatherapists could take a massive workload away from the doctor's surgeries.

- Discover the hormonal changes and peptide triggers that change a person's health and mental state.
- Learn how it affects the liver, adrenals and pituitary gland.
- Uncover the strange phenomenon of Yin disease

- Build a better foundation of care, but also a knowledge base that means you can sell your treatments more effectively.
- Improve your healing skills set
- Supercharge your referrals potential from other complementary therapists and orthodox medicine alike.

Includes free bonus material of

- Chiropractic chart of misalignments and potential organic disturbance
- Chart of the meridians and suggested acupressure points to detox the organs more quickly
- Detailed information about how to improve the patients condition with vitamin and minerals therapy
- In depth dietary advice
- Free hypnotherapy relaxation download

Essential Oils are The Off Switch for stress. The *Professional Stress Solution* is the ON SWITCH for your aromatherapy business.

Book 5 The Aromatherapy Eczema Treatment

Healing Eczema, Itchy Skin Rashes and Atopic Dermatitis with Essential Oils and Holistic Medicine

Most people appreciate that the itching and redness of eczema can be used using essential oils, but what if I told you they were capable of so much more?

Imagine if, as a therapist, you were able to pinpoint the emotions that set off these flares? Can you visualise what it would mean to your patient if you were able to isolate the very protagonist causing the eczema breakout and alleviate their pain completely?

Well now you can.

This book teaches you:

- How to isolate the emotions causing the emotional cycle of pain
- The likely food triggers for your patient and the tools to identify the exact times they will detonate a reaction
- The familial traits and links that lead to atopic eczema
- How these links connect with the liver and in turn how to cleanse the liver toxicity
- Vitamins and minerals to cleanse and nourish the system

The book contains very real that will not only transform the way you treat clients, but will skyrocket your clinic's takings.

I recommend reading this book in tandem with *The Professional Stress Solution* and the *Essential Oil Liver Cleanse* to fully understand the cycles and processes of treatment. Add to it *Sales Strategies for Gentle Souls* and your business will stand on an entirely new footing.

Why not save yourself 1/3

And treat yourself to the set?

The full and comprehensive course into how to heal eczema

with aromatherapy and essential oils I promise you...nothing else comes even close.

Sales Strategies for Gentle Souls

Targeted Sales Training for Professional Aromatherapists

Wonderful things are happening in complementary therapy. Very gifted people are churning out fantastic research and results. The internet is full of what essential oils can do. But when a gentle soul emerges from their relaxing haze of their aromatherapy class room, how do they harness the buzz of energy around them for their craft?

From 1999-2008 I worked in one of the most aggressive commercial environments there is. My role as a recruitment consultant was 80% cold calling in am extremely saturated sales arena. Despite my own gentle soul, I found ways not only to compete, but to excel.

- Learn how to pinpoint the best customers for your practice
- Cost your treatments to ensure every treatment is profitable for both you and your customer
- Discover how to make every conversation into a potential sale lead without becoming a complete and utter pain in the a*s!
- Uncover the reasons why you are not closing sales so you never have to make the same mistakes again
- Create a growth environment where you plan success and always find yourself stepping into it

If you are working with essential oils, and you want to make a good living for it, then you need to learn to sell. What's more, if you are going to say "selling doesn't work on my customers"….then you have simply been taught to do it wrongly.

My dream is to see aromatherapy at the forefront of medicine. I need an army of gifted healers to achieve that. Consider yourself to be my newest recruit and I am going to drill you till you are the slickest, subtlest and most effective marketeer there is. You have the knowledge to make people better, now let me give you the business prowess to heal even more people than you have ever done before.

The Secret Healer has stress in her sights and she's about to make a killing. Listen carefully...she has much to tell you.

www.thesecrethealer.co.uk

www.buildyourownreality.com

Bibliography

Amestejani M1, S. B. (2007). *Vitamin D supplementation in the treatment of atopic dermatitis: a clinical trial study.* Retrieved 07 28, 2014, from National Library of medicine: http://www.ncbi.nlm.nih.gov/pubmed/22395583

Anderson C1, L.-B. M.-S. (2000, 09 20). *Evaluation of massage with essential oils on childhood atopic eczema.* Retrieved 07 28, 2014, from National Library of Medicine: http://umm.edu/health/medical/altmed/condition/eczema

Bruce, J. (1995). Advanced Aromatherapy Diploma. *Jill Bruce School of Aromatherapy* .

Bruce, J. *The Garden of Eden.*

Centre, U. o. (n.d.). *Eczema.* Retrieved 07 28, 2014, from University of Maryland Medical Centre: http://umm.edu/health/medical/altmed/condition/eczema

E Van Epps, G. H. (Mar , 1976;). Liver disease--a prominent cause of serum IgE elevation. *Clin Exp Immunol.* , pp. 23(3): 444-450.

Enzymatic profile, adhesive and invasive properties of Candida albicans under the influence of selected plant essential oils. (2014). Retrieved 07 28, 2014, from Budzyńska

A, Sadowska B, Więckowska-Szakiel M, Różalska B.: http://www.ncbi.nlm.nih.gov/pubmed/24644554

Ernst E1, P. M. (2002). *Complementary/alternative medicine in dermatology: evidence-assessed efficacy of two diseases and two treatments.* Retrieved 2014, from National Library of Medicine: http://www.ncbi.nlm.nih.gov/pubmed/12069640

Fischer, K. (2012). *The Eczema Diet.* Exisle Publishing.

Functions of Acid Mantle. (2012). Retrieved 7 28, 2014, from Docté Botanical Research: http://www.docte.net/your_skin/skin_knowledge/acid_mantle.php

Giarratana F1, M. D. (2014, 07). *Activity of Thymus vulgaris essential oil against Anisakis larvae.* Retrieved 07 2014, from http://www.ncbi.nlm.nih.gov/pubmed/24721259

H Kimata: Department of Pediatrics and Allergy, U. H. (2005). *Prevalence of fatty liver in non-obese Japanese children with atopic dermatitis.* Retrieved 7 28, 2014, from National Library of Medicine: http://www.ncbi.nlm.nih.gov/pubmed/15995275

Hariya T1, K. Y. (2002). *Effects of sedative odorant inhalation on patients with atopic dermatitis.* Retrieved from National Library of Medicine: http://www.ncbi.nlm.nih.gov/pubmed/12486337

Hederos CA1, B. A. (1996). *Epogam evening primrose oil treatment in atopic dermatitis and asthma.* Retrieved 07 28, 2014, from National Library of medicine: http://www.ncbi.nlm.nih.gov/pubmed/9014601

James M Mason, 1. J. (2013, 5 16). *Improved emollient use reduces atopic eczema symptoms and is cost neutral in infants: before-and-after evaluation of a multifaceted educational support programme.* Retrieved 7 28, 2014, from National Library of Medicine: http://www.ncbi.nlm.nih.gov/pmc/articles/PMC3665665/

Janmejai K Srivastava, E. S. (2010, 11 10). *Chamomile: A herbal medicine of the past with bright future.* Retrieved 07 28, 2014, from National Library of Medicine: http://www.ncbi.nlm.nih.gov/pmc/articles/PMC2995283/

Jones, J. B. (2003). *Efficacy and tolerability of borage oil in adults and children with atopic eczema: randomised, double blind, placebo controlled, parallel group trial.* Retrieved 2014, from British Medical Journal: http://www.bmj.com/content/327/7428/1385?ijkey=851d1ee4929b96e779d52b9f703b25a3e4733092&keytype2=tf_ipsecsha

Judith Hong, M. J. (2011, 06). *Management of Itch in Atopic Dermatitis.* Retrieved 07 28, 2014, from National Library of

Medicine: http://www.ncbi.nlm.nih.gov/pmc/articles/PMC3704137/

Kanehara S1, O. T. (2007). *Clinical effects of undershirts coated with borage oil on children with atopic dermatitis: a double-blind, placebo-controlled clinical trial.* Retrieved 07 28, 2014, from National Library of Medicine: http://www.ncbi.nlm.nih.gov/pubmed/18078406

Kerscher MJ1, K. H.-M. (1992). *Treatment of atopic eczema with evening primrose oil: rationale and clinical results.* Retrieved 7 28, 2014, from National Libraries of Medicine: http://www.ncbi.nlm.nih.gov/pubmed/1318129

Lancet. (1998). *Worldwide variation in prevalence of symptoms of asthma, allergic rhinoconjunctivitis, and atopic eczema: ISAAC. The International Study of Asthma and Allergies in Childhood (ISAAC) Steering Committee.* Retrieved 7 28, 2014, from US National Library of Medicine: http://www.ncbi.nlm.nih.gov/pubmed/9643741

Lee KC1, K. A. (2012, 03). *Effectiveness of acupressure on pruritus and lichenification associated with atopic dermatitis: a pilot trial.* Retrieved 07 28, 2014, from National Library of Medicine: http://www.ncbi.nlm.nih.gov/pubmed/22207450

Lynn M.Taussig, M. A. (n.d.). *Tucson Children's Respiratory Study: 1980 to Present.* Retrieved 7 28, 2014, from Current reviews of allergy and clinical immunology: http://www.cercnotti.com.ar/archivos/postgrado/ASMA-FENOTIP-TUCSON-HT-HOY.pdf

M C Arrieta, L. B. (n.d.). *Alterations of Intestinal permeability.* Retrieved 7 28, 2014, from International Journal of Gastroenterology and Hepatology: http://www.ncbi.nlm.nih.gov/pmc/articles/PMC1856434/

M.I. Asher, U. K. (1995). *International study of asthma and allergies in childhood (ISAAC):.* Retrieved 7 28, 2014, from European Respiratory Journal: http://erj.ersjournals.com/content/8/3/483.full.pdf

Manso. (2014). *Eczema.* Retrieved 7 28, 2014, from The Whole Health Centre: http://drmanso.com/patient-education-guide/eczema/

Medicine, S. S. (201). *Food Allergies FAQ Symptoms, Testing and Therapies.* Retrieved 07 28, 2014, from Stanford School of Medicine- Food Allergies Division: http://foodallergies.stanford.edu/learn/food-allergy-faq.html#one

Michael J. Cork, P. F.-A. (2006, 03). *New perspectives on epidermal barrier dysfunction in atopic dermatitis: Gene–*

environment interactions. Retrieved 7 28, 2014, from The Journal of Allergy and Clinical Immunology: http://www.jacionline.org/article/S0091-6749(06)00935-3/abstract

Myhill, S. (2012, 1 13). *Nutritional deficiencies - What signs to look for if you think you may have them.* Retrieved 7 28, 2014, from Dr Myhill: http://www.drmyhill.co.uk/wiki/Nutritional_deficiencies_-_What_signs_to_look_for_if_you_think_you_may_have_them

PD., S. (2003). *Biofeedback, cognitive-behavioral methods, and hypnosis in dermatology: is it all in your mind?* Retrieved 2014, from National Library of medicine: http://www.ncbi.nlm.nih.gov/pubmed/12919113

PD., S. (2000). *Hypnosis in dermatology.* Retrieved 2014, from National Libraryof Medicine: http://www.ncbi.nlm.nih.gov/pubmed/10724204

Pommier P1, G. F. (2004). *Phase III randomized trial of Calendula officinalis compared with trolamine for the prevention of acute dermatitis during irradiation for breast cancer.* Retrieved 07 28, 2014, from National Library of Medicine: http://www.ncbi.nlm.nih.gov/pubmed/15084618

Savolainen J1, L. K. (1993, 04). *Candida albicans and atopic dermatitis*. Retrieved 07 28, 2014, from LIbrary of Medicine: http://www.ncbi.nlm.nih.gov/pubmed/8319131

Shimelis ND1, A. S. (2012). *Researching accessible and affordable treatment for common dermatological problems in developing countries. An Ethiopian experience.* Retrieved 07 28, 2014, from National Library o fMedicine: http://www.ncbi.nlm.nih.gov/pubmed/22715822

Swapan Senapati, S. B. (2008). *Evening primrose oil is effective in atopic dermatitis: A randomized placebo-controlled trial.* Retrieved 07 28, 2014, from Indian Journal of Dermatology, Venerealogy and Leprology: http://www.ijdvl.com/article.asp?issn=0378-6323;year=2008;volume=74;issue=5;spage=447;epage=452;aulast=Senapati

Tao Zheng Jinho Yu, M. H. (2011, Apr). *The Atopic March: Progression from Atopic Dermatitis to Allergic Rhinitis and Asthma.* Retrieved Jul 11, 2014, from Allergy Asthma Immunol Res (3/2): http://www.ncbi.nlm.nih.gov/pmc/articles/PMC3062798/

Types of Eczema. (2014). Retrieved 07 28, 2014, from National Society of Eczema: http://www.eczema.org/types-of-eczema

Werdin González JO1, L. R. (2013, 07). *Lethal and sublethal effects of four essential oils on the egg parasitoids Trissolcus basalis.* Retrieved 07 28, 2014, from National Library of Medicine: http://www.ncbi.nlm.nih.gov/pubmed/23664473

Williams, H. C. (2003). *Evening Primrose for Atopic Dermatitis.* Retrieved 07 28, 2014, from British Medical Journal: http://www.bmj.com/content/327/7428/1358

Worward, V. A. *The Fragrant Pharmacy.*

Worwood, V. A. *The Fragrant Mind.*

Yunes Panahi, 1. ,. (2012). *A Randomized Comparative Trial on the Therapeutic Efficacy of Topical Aloe vera and Calendula officinalis on Diaper Dermatitis in Children.* Retrieved 7 28, 2014, from National Library of Medicine: http://www.ncbi.nlm.nih.gov/pmc/articles/PMC3346674/

Zore GB1, T. A. (2011). *Evaluation of anti-Candida potential of geranium oil constituents against clinical isolates of Candida albicans differentially sensitive to fluconazole: inhibition of growth, dimorphism and sensitization.* Retrieved 07 2014, from National Library of Medicine: http://www.ncbi.nlm.nih.gov/pubmed/20337938

Disclaimer

by SEQ Legal

(1)   Introduction

This disclaimer governs the use of this book. [By using this book, you accept this disclaimer in full. / We will ask you to agree to this disclaimer before you can access the book.]

(2)   Credit

This disclaimer was created using an SEQ Legal template.

(3)   No advice

The book contains information about aromatherapy and the use of essential oils. The information is not advice, and should not be treated as such.

[You must not rely on the information in the book as an alternative to qualified medical advice from a health professional. advice from an appropriately qualified professional. If you have any specific questions about any medical matter you should consult an appropriately qualified professional.]

[If you think you may be suffering from any medical condition you should seek immediate medical attention. You should never delay seeking medical advice, disregard medical advice, or discontinue medical treatment because of information in the book.]

(4)   No representations or warranties

To the maximum extent permitted by applicable law and subject to section 6 below, we exclude all representations, warranties, undertakings and guarantees relating to the book.

Without prejudice to the generality of the foregoing paragraph, we do not represent, warrant, undertake or guarantee:

> that the information in the book is correct, accurate, complete or non-misleading;

> that the use of the guidance in the book will lead to any particular outcome or result; or

> in particular, that by using the guidance in the book you will heal disease or work in any way as a cure for illness.

(5) Limitations and exclusions of liability

The limitations and exclusions of liability set out in this section and elsewhere in this disclaimer: are subject to section 6 below; and govern all liabilities arising under the disclaimer or in relation to the book, including liabilities arising in contract, in tort (including negligence) and for breach of statutory duty.

We will not be liable to you in respect of any losses arising out of any event or events beyond our reasonable control.

We will not be liable to you in respect of any business losses, including without limitation loss of or damage to profits, income, revenue, use, production, anticipated savings, business, contracts, commercial opportunities or goodwill.

We will not be liable to you in respect of any loss or corruption of any data, database or software.

We will not be liable to you in respect of any special, indirect or consequential loss or damage.

(6) Exceptions

Nothing in this disclaimer shall: limit or exclude our liability for death or personal injury resulting from negligence; limit or exclude our liability for fraud or fraudulent misrepresentation; limit any of our liabilities in any way that is not permitted under applicable law; or exclude any of our liabilities that may not be excluded under applicable law.

(7) Severability

If a section of this disclaimer is determined by any court or other competent authority to be unlawful and/or unenforceable, the other sections of this disclaimer continue in effect.

If any unlawful and/or unenforceable section would be lawful or enforceable if part of it were deleted, that part will be deemed to be deleted, and the rest of the section will continue in effect.

(8) Law and jurisdiction

This disclaimer will be governed by and construed in accordance with English law, and any disputes relating to this disclaimer will be subject to the exclusive jurisdiction of the courts of England and Wales.

(9) Our details

In this disclaimer, "we" means (and "us" and "our" refer to) The Secret Healer / buildyourownreality.com, a partnership established under English law having its principal place of business at 4, SY8 1LQ.

So what is eczema?

Back up iGe related to liver dysfunction. http://www.ncbi.nlm.nih.gov/pmc/articles/PMC1538400/

http://connection.ebscohost.com/c/articles/78348527/evaluation-serum-igg-igm-iga-ige-levels-patients-chronic-liver-diseases

http://www.unboundmedicine.com/medline/citation/7584688/Increased_serum_IgE_in_alcohol_abusers_

https://wao.confex.com/wao/2011wac/webprogram/Paper4114.html

Printed in Great Britain
by Amazon.co.uk, Ltd.,
Marston Gate.